MCQs in Medicine for MI

MCQs in Medicine for MRCP Part 1

Andrew Provan
MB ChB MRCP
Registrar, Department of Haematology,
Stobhill Hospital, Glasgow

CHURCHILL LIVINGSTONE
EDINBURGH LONDON MELBOURNE AND NEW YORK 1990

CHURCHILL LIVINGSTONE
Medical Division of Longman Group UK Limited

Distributed in the United States of America by Churchill Livingstone Inc., 1560 Broadway, New York, N.Y. 10036, and by associated companies, branches and representatives throughout the world.

© Longman Group UK Limited 1990

All rights reserved. No part of this publication may be reproduced, stored in a retrieval system, or transmitted in any form or by any means, electronic, mechanical, photocopying, recording or otherwise, without either the prior written permission of the publishers (Churchill Livingstone, Robert Stevenson House, 1–3 Baxter's Place, Leith Walk, Edinburgh EH1 3AF), or a licence permitting restricted copying in the United Kingdom issued by the Copyright Licensing Agency Ltd, 33–34 Alfred Place, London, WC1E 7DP.

First published 1990

ISBN 0-443-04220-9

British Library Cataloguing in Publication Data
Provan, Andrew
  MCQs in Medicine for MRCP Part 1.
  1. Medicine
  I. Title
  610

Produced by Longman Singapore Publishers (Pte) Ltd.
Printed in Singapore

Preface

Obtaining the MRCP qualification is much easier said than done. It is a major career milestone for physicians in training and for many can be a soul-destroying experience. (For a description of the examination philosophy and format see 'MRCP 1977' British Medical Journal 1978, 1:217.) People vary in their approaches to Parts 1 and 2 and obviously there is no *single* way to work. In an exam which is competitive and has a high rate of failure and of which the Part 1 is an example, it pays to maximise your chances by planning your time carefully and preparing, not in a way which encompasses the whole of medicine, but in a way which prepares you for this specific exam. Many people, although widely-read and apparently very knowledgeable, fail this exam because of either lack of preparation or poor technique in answering MCQs.

Some 10 years ago there were few books aimed at helping candidates over this hurdle but fortunately this has changed and there are now several MCQ books on the market. The justification, therefore, for this book's joining the list is that part of the key to passing this exam is practice: the more practised a candidate is at answering this form of question, the less likely it is that he or she will be taken unawares in the real exam. If I have any advice at all for prospective MRCP candidates it would be to practise as many questions as you can get hold of. Once these have been completed, start again! In a sense one can 'learn' the questions. By practising MCQs candidates will get to know their weaker areas and can concentrate on these before sitting the real examination.

I would suggest using this book some 6 weeks or so before the exam and after trying the MCQs in a section some further reading could be done and notes made from the information obtained. Candidates should read their own notes as often as possible to 'imprint' the information, since they then will be able to recall it more easily later.

Although this book of MCQs is aimed primarily at the junior doctor working for MRCP Part 1, it should also be of interest to final year medical students who meet MCQs in General Medicine as part of the finals examinations.

vi PREFACE

I hope these questions are of value. The reading list, although not extensive, is one that I personally found useful.

Good luck!

Glasgow, 1989   A.P.

Acknowledgements

I would like to thank various colleagues who have read and made comments on the manuscript; in particular I am grateful to Drs Peter Dawes and Michael Gavin for their helpful suggestions. Thanks are due also to Churchill Livingstone for their support and for taking on this project in the first place. Most of all I would like to thank my wife, Val, for all her help and encouragement.

Contents

How to use this book	x
1. Basic sciences (Questions 1–40)	1
2. Cardiology (Questions 1–30)	17
3. Dermatology (Questions 1–10)	29
4. Endocrinology (Questions 1–20)	33
5. Gastroenterology (Questions 1–20)	41
6. Genetics (Questions 1–5)	49
7. Haematology (Questions 1–25)	51
8. Infectious/tropical diseases (Questions 1–25)	61
9. Metabolic disease (Questions 1–20)	71
10. Neurology (Questions 1–20)	79
11. Ophthalmology (Questions 1–5)	87
12. Paediatrics (Questions 1–15)	89
13. Pharmacology (Questions 1–25)	95
14. Renal disease (Questions 1–20)	105
15. Respiratory medicine (Questions 1–20)	113
16. Rheumatology/immunology (Questions 1–20)	121
17. Statistics (Questions 1–5)	129
Recommended reading	133
Index	137

How to use this book

The text consists of questions on the right-hand page with their corresponding answers overleaf on a left-hand page.

Any number of the statements in each question may be correct.

1. Basic sciences

1. **Regarding sodium homeostasis:**
   a. oedema states are associated with an increase in total body sodium
   b. diet usually provides about 1500 mmol/24 hours
   c. sodium is reabsorbed passively in the ascending limb of the loop of Henle
   d. total body sodium is about 5000 mmol
   e. sodium loading has a minor effect on aldosterone secretion

2. **The following statements about plasma proteins are correct:**
   a. haptoglobin is an α-2 globulin
   b. transferrin levels rise in iron deficiency
   c. fibrinogen is one of the globulins
   d. α-1 antitrypsin inhibits pepsin
   e. transferrin is an α-2 globulin

3. **The following statements about vitamins and minerals are true:**
   a. vitamin A is transported bound to albumin
   b. riboflavin is fat-soluble
   c. a high concentration of vitamin C is found in the thymus and pituitary gland
   d. growth and sexual development retardation are features of zinc deficiency
   e. molybdenum has not been recognised as an essential element in man

4. **Bile acid functions include:**
   a. absorption of water-soluble vitamins from the gut
   b. inhibition of pancreatic lipase
   c. decrease in colonic motility
   d. solubilisation of cholesterol
   e. enhanced water and electrolyte absorption by the large bowel

(Answers overleaf)

2 MCQS IN MEDICINE FOR MRCP PART 1

1 a c d
(margin note: intake of Na⁺ <1500mg)
Total body sodium rises due to relative hypovolaemia ± poor cardiac function. These promote renin release and hence hyperaldosteronism which results in Na^+ retention. Diet provides ≈150 mmol Na^+/day and Na^+ loading has a major effect on aldosterone secretion. *(handwritten: ↑Na⁺ - ↑blood pressure - ↓RAA ie. ↓aldosterone)*

2 a b c
Haptoglobin is an α-2 globulin which binds haemoglobin from damaged red blood cells. Transferrin is a β-globulin of molecular weight 90 000. α-1 antitrypsin inhibits trypsin, plasmin and chymotrypsin.

3 a c d
Riboflavin is water-soluble. Molybdenum, like chromium, selenium and vanadium, is an essential element in man.

4 b d
Bile acids aid the absorption of fat-soluble vitamins, increase colonic motility and decrease water and electrolyte absorption in the large bowel. They also inhibit pancreatic lipase and increase secretion of phospholipid.

(handwritten notes at bottom:)
Fat soluble = A, D, E, K

Zinc deficiency — skin ulcer, ↓ immune system, hypogondal dwarfism

5 **Adrenocorticotrophic hormone (ACTH):**
   a is a steroid hormone
   b is derived from β-endorphin
   c is secreted in response to noise
   d has a half-life of 2 hours
   e induces ketosis

6 **Factors which cause the oxygen dissociation curve to shift to the right include:**
   a increase in hydrogen ion concentration
   b increase in carbon dioxide concentration
   c decrease in temperature
   d increase in 2,3-DPG
   e fetal haemoglobin

7 **The following statements about radial nerve palsy are true:**
   a arsenic poisoning is a recognised cause
   b extension at the elbow is lost if the lesion occurs distal to the triceps innervation
   c shoulder dislocation is a recognised cause
   d in a complete palsy the triceps reflex is lost
   e palsies induced by pressure on the nerve do not result in muscular atrophy

8 **The diaphragm:**
   a has an opening for the aorta and thoracic duct at T10 level
   b is formed by fusion of the septum transversum, dorsal oesophageal mesentery and pleuropericardial membranes
   c has all its sensory nerve supply from the lower intercostal nerves
   d has an opening for the inferior vena cava at T8 level
   e has a central tendon which is fused to the anterior pericardium

9 **The following statements about the lumbo-sacral plexus are correct:**
   a it originates from the posterior primary rami of L1-S4
   b the obturator nerve supplies the gracilis muscle
   c the femoral nerve is derived from L1-4
   d the saphenous nerve supplies sensation to the medial side of the leg
   e the superior gluteal nerve has the root value L5, S1-2

(Answers overleaf)

5 c
ACTH is a polypeptide of 39 amino acids. It controls secretion of cortisol by the adrenal cortex and increases blood flow through the adrenal glands. Stimulators of release include hypoglycaemia, circadian rhythm, exercise and emotional stress. Its half life is 10 minutes and its actions are mediated via cAMP. It is derived, along with pro-MSH and β-LPH, from pro-opiocortin.

6 a b d
Increased affinity of haemoglobin for oxygen (curve shifted to the *left*) is caused by carbon monoxide poisoning, massive blood transfusion and fetal haemoglobin. The affinity of haemoglobin for oxygen is reduced (curve shifted to the *right*) by rising pCO_2 levels, acidosis, increased temperature and increased levels of 2,3-DPG.

7 a c d e
The radial nerve is derived from C6-8 and T1 and is the largest branch of the brachial plexus. Palsies may occur due to trauma (fracture of humerus and shoulder dislocation), pressure ('Saturday night palsy') and toxins such as lead and arsenic. Complete palsy will lead to extensor paralysis with pronation of the hand and wrist drop. Lesions occurring below that of triceps innervation do not result in loss of extension at the elbow. Sensory loss is minimal. Muscle atrophy is apparently absent in palsies induced by pressure.

8 b d
The diaphragm is made up of two portions: the outer muscular part and a central tendon. Its nerve supply is from C3,4,5. The peripheral intercostal nerves supply sensation to the peripheral diaphragm. There are three openings: one for the aorta (at T12), one for the oesophagus (at T10) and the third for the inferior vena cava (at T8). The central tendon is partially fused to the undersurface of the pericardium.

9 b c d
The lumbosacral plexus is derived from the anterior primary rami of L1-S4. The superior gluteal nerve has the root value L4-5,S1

BASIC SCIENCES

10 The following are true of the tenth cranial nerve (vagus):
  a sensory fibres originate in the nucleus ambiguus
  b postganglionic parasympathetic fibres inhibit adrenal gland secretion
  c diphtheria is a recognised cause of peripheral lesions of the tenth cranial nerve
  d bilateral vagal paralysis is associated with gastric dilatation
  e both vagi enter the abdominal cavity by passing through the aortic opening in the diaphragm

11 Excitatory neurotransmitters in the central nervous system include:
  a acetylcholine
  b dopamine
  c glutamate
  d gamma-aminobutyric acid (GABA)
  e substance P

12 Increased renal excretion of magnesium occurs with:
  a alcoholism
  b thyroxine
  c metabolic acidosis
  d glucagon
  e respiratory acidosis

13 Causes of a raised creatine kinase include:
  a polymyositis
  b hypothyroidism
  c pulmonary infarction
  d leukaemia
  e liver disease

14 The following statements are true:
  a serum immunoglobulin levels are higher in African negroes than Caucasians
  b serum albumin is lower in the erect position than the supine position
  c serum creatine kinase is higher in males
  d serum lactate dehydrogenase levels are higher than normal in serum if blood is left standing at room temperature for 1 hour
  e serum vitamin D levels show a seasonal variation

15 The following, if found in conjunction with a paraproteinaemia, suggest malignancy:
  a Bence Jones protein at a concentration of <1 g/l
  b immune paresis
  c presence of IgD paraproteinaemia
  d IgG in a concentration of 5 g/l
  e increasing paraprotein level.

(Answers overleaf)

10 b c d
The vagus has motor, parasympathetic, somatic and visceral sensory fibres. Motor fibres originate in the nucleus ambiguus. Complete bilateral palsies of the tenth cranial nerve lead to laryngeal paralysis, aphonia, dilatation of the stomach, cardiac arrhythmias and death. In unilateral lesions there is unilateral soft palate paralysis, hoarseness and dysphagia. The vagi enter the abdomen by passing through the oesophageal opening in the diaphragm.

11 a c e
Acetylcholine has both excitatory and inhibitory actions in the CNS. The mono-amines are basically inhibitory and these include dopamine, 5HT, noradrenaline and adrenaline. Glutamate and aspartate are excitatory amino acid neurotransmitters. Glycine and GABA are both inhibitory.

12 a b c
High serum magnesium is associated with renal failure, burns and diabetic ketoacidosis. Alcoholics are prone to hypomagnesaemia due to poor diet and increased renal excretion of magnesium due to the diuretic state which is produced. Alkalosis promotes increased movement of magnesium into cells and insulin promotes urinary magnesium excretion. Glucagon and respiratory acidosis result in decreased magnesium excretion.

13 a b c
Creatine kinase is found in heart, skeletal muscle and brain. Elevation of serum levels may be due to polymyositis, myocardial infarction, muscular dystrophies, hypothyroidism, trauma, alcoholism and pulmonary infarction.

14 a c d e
Serum albumin levels are higher in the erect position. Vitamin D levels show a seasonal variation reflecting the different levels of sun exposure.

15 b c e
Those features suggesting malignancy include Bence Jones proteinaemia of ≥1 g/l and IgG at 20 g/l. IgD and IgE proteinaemia are always malignant. Immune paresis and an increasing paraprotein level are highly suggestive of malignancy.

BASIC SCIENCES

16 The following statements relating to prostaglandin (PG) metabolism are true:
   a cyclo-oxygenase (COX) is inhibited by glucocorticoids
   b arachidonic acid is converted to hydroperoxy acids by lipoxygenase (LOX)
   c PGE_2 promotes contraction of smooth muscle
   d thromboxane A_2 acts by inhibition of adenyl cyclase
   e PGI_2 is derived from leukotriene A_4

17 Haemodialysis is better than peritoneal dialysis for elimination of:
   a ethylene glycol
   b barbiturates
   c isopropanol
   d lithium
   e disopyramide

18 The following statements are true:
   a blood pressure is maintained by receptors situated in the aortic arch
   b peripheral resistance in blood vessels is the product of cardiac output and mean arterial pressure
   c increase in afferent traffic in the IX and X cranial nerves leads to a response in baroreceptors in the carotid sinus
   d mean portal vein pressure is around 30 mmHg
   e bradykinin has no role in maintaining the calibre of arterial vessels

19 Somatomedin:
   a is synthesised in the pituitary
   b has a half life of 20 minutes
   c acts with growth hormone to promote growth
   d is a steroid hormone
   e is lipolytic

20 Factors promoting gastrin release include:
   a secretin
   b pernicious anaemia
   c small bowel resection
   d atropine
   e ethanol

21 The ulnar nerve:
   a has the root value C6-8
   b supplies adductor pollicis
   c arises from the lateral cord of the brachial plexus
   d supplies all the hypothenar muscles
   e supplies abductor pollicis longus

(Answers overleaf)

steroid *phospholipid*
Phospholipase A2 ⟶ ↓
                   arachidonic acid

16 b c d
Arachidonic acid has a central role in prostaglandin synthesis. From it, leukotrienes are synthesised (via lipoxygenase) and endoperoxides are made via cyclo-oxygenase. Cyclo-oxygenase is inhibited by non-steroidal anti-inflammatory drugs and PGI_2 is derived from PGG_2, an endoperoxide. The leukotrienes are a separate group of compounds.

17 a c d
Haemodialysis is better than peritoneal dialysis for the elimination of methanol, isopropanol, lithium and ethylene glycol. Barbiturate toxicity is better dealt with by haemoperfusion as is disopyramide overdose.

18 a c
Arterial blood pressure is maintained by neural and humoral mechanisms. The neural system comprises receptors in the aortic arch and carotid sinus which respond to rises and falls in blood pressure. The humoral system acts via the renin-angiotensin system to maintain blood pressure.

Peripheral resistance = arterial pressure ÷ cardiac output.

Mean portal pressure is ≈ 10 mmHg. Bradykinin, along with pCO_2 and pO_2, catecholamines, angiotensin and glucocorticoids, determines the calibre of resistance vessels.

19 c
growth factors e.g. insulin like growth factor-1, rll, relaxin
Somatomedin is synthesised in the <u>liver</u> and has a $t\frac{1}{2}$ of several hours. It is a polypeptide and has antilipolytic actions.

20 b c e
secretion affected by
1) stomach content
2) vagus nerve
3) Blood-borne factors
Gastrin is a polypeptide of 34 amino acids and is secreted by the G cells of the stomach and duodenum. It stimulates water and acid secretion by the stomach and increases gastric blood flow. Factors promoting release include: antral distension, (*after eating*) *protein* *A vagal discharge* Ca^{2+} catecholamines, low dose ethanol and meat meals. Those factors which prevent gastrin release include secretin, (atropine) and antral acidification. — *gastric acid* GIP calcitonin
somatostatin VIP
                glucagon

21 b d
The ulnar nerve (C7-8,T1) is derived from the medial cord of the brachial plexus. It supplies branches to flexor carpi ulnaris, the medial half of flexor digitorum profundus, the hypothenar muscles, interossei, third and fourth lumbricals and adductor pollicis. It supplies cutaneous sensation to the ulnar aspect of the hand and both surfaces of the ulnar 1½ fingers.

- 2 muscles in forearm
- nerve of fine movements
- Innervates intrinsic muscle concerned with intricate hand movements.

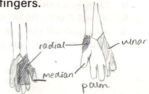

BASIC SCIENCES

22 The following statements about the anatomy of the heart are correct:
  a the left atrium is larger than the right
  b the anterior mitral valve leaflet is larger than the posterior
  c most of the venous drainage of the heart is via venae cordis directly into the cardiac cavity
  d arterial supply via the marginal branch is derived from the left anterior descending coronary artery
  e cervical sympathetic ganglia form part of the nerve supply of the heart

23 Substances activating muscarinic cholinergic receptors include:
  a methacholine
  b pilocarpine
  c acetylcholine
  d neostigmine
  e tetramethylammonium

24 The following statements about histamine are correct:
  a platelets are a rich source of histamine
  b L-histidine decarboxylase is involved in histamine breakdown
  c histamine is found in both animals and plants
  d its actions include capillary dilatation
  e synergism is seen between histamine and beer

25 The following statements about respiration before and after birth are true:
  a amniotic fluid is absorbed by the lungs of the fetus
  b respiratory movements are first seen at about 30 weeks' gestation
  c in the neonate the vital capacity is ≈50–100 ml
  d the functional residual capacity of the neonate is 75 ml
  e the tidal volume of a newborn baby is around 500 ml

26 Reabsorption of phosphate by the kidneys is increased in:
  a hypercalcaemia
  b patients on a low phosphate diet
  c alcoholism
  d an alkaline urine
  e insulin treatment

27 Serum ferritin levels rise in:
  a hepatoma
  b primary haemochromatosis
  c iron deficiency
  d carcinoma
  e pregnancy

(Answers overleaf)

22 b e

The left atrium is smaller than the right but is thicker-walled. The anterior leaflet of the mitral valve is larger than the posterior. Two thirds of the venous drainage of the heart is by veins accompanying the coronary arteries, which drain into the right atrium. The rest is by venae cordis which drain directly into the cardiac cavity. The marginal branch is derived from the right coronary artery and the nerve supply is from the cervical and thoracic sympathetic ganglia along with the vagus.

23 a b c

Methacholine has muscarinic effects which are most obvious in the cardiovascular system (affects atrial tissue and has been used in the treatment of supraventricular tachycardia). Pilocarpine is used in glaucoma because of its actions as pupillary constrictor. Acetylcholine has muscarinic *and* nicotinic actions including contraction of bladder muscle, constriction of the pupil, gut contraction and penile erection. Neostigmine and tetramethylammonium have nicotinic effects.

24 c d

Histamine is a biogenic amine found in mast cells, basophils and gastric mucosa. L-histidine decarboxylase is involved in its *synthesis* and breakdown occurs in most tissues of the body. It causes constriction of bronchioles, uterine contraction, capillary relaxation and hypotension. CNS depression is marked if antihistamines are taken with alcohol.

25 a c

Before birth the amniotic fluid is absorbed by the fetal lungs. Respiratory movements are seen from about 12 weeks' gestation. After birth the specific gravity of the lungs falls and the respiratory rate is around 30 per minute. Tidal volume is about 17 ml and dead space 5 ml. The FRC is 75 ml.

26 a b e

The renal threshold for phosphate reabsorption is largely dependent upon parathyroid hormone (PTH). If the PTH concentration rises then phosphate reabsorption is decreased. Renal phosphate reabsorption is also decreased in patients on high phosphate diets, diuretics or thyroxine and in alcoholics. Renal phosphate reabsorption is increased in patients who are on insulin therapy, have increased growth hormone levels and are on low phosphate diets.

27 a b d

Ferritin is a water-soluble protein-iron complex (cf haemosiderin which is water-insoluble) and is a storage form of iron. Ferritin levels are high in the newborn, haemochromatosis, malignancy, paracetamol poisoning, liver disease and hepatoma. Levels are reduced in pregnancy and iron deficiency.

BASIC SCIENCES

28 Clinical features of hypokalaemia include:
  a hyperchloraemia
  b metabolic acidosis
  c increase in aldosterone secretion
  d polyuria
  e ileus

29 The following are recognised causes of nephrogenic diabetes insipidus:
  a myeloma
  b polycystic kidney disease
  c chlorpropamide
  d demeclocycline
  e analgesic nephropathy

30 Parathyroid hormone:
  a increases renal tubular reabsorption of phosphate
  b stimulates osteoblastic activity
  c actions are antagonised by calcitonin secreted by the parathyroid glands
  d elevates plasma free ionised calcium
  e action on bone is impaired in the absence of 1,25-dihydroxycholecalciferol

31 Proteinuria:
  a if orthostatic is more marked in the supine position
  b in 'normal' people may be up to 0.08 g/day
  c if tubular in origin is predominantly albumin
  d if glomerular is usually <1 g/day
  e of the Bence Jones variety will give a false-positive result on stick testing ('Albustix')

32 The following are recognised causes of hypomagnesaemia:
  a diabetes mellitus
  b chronic diarrhoea
  c hypothyroidism
  d burns
  e chronic hypercapnia

(Answers overleaf)

28 d e
Hypokalaemia may lead to weakness and paralysis of skeletal muscle as well as intestinal ileus. Polyuria and polydipsia are features, as are hyponatraemia and chloride wasting. Metabolic *alkalosis* rather than acidosis occurs.

29 a b d e
Diabetes insipidus may be central (pituitary surgery, tumour, trauma, sarcoidosis, histiocytosis X, etc) or nephrogenic. The latter may be congenital or acquired. Drugs which cause it include glibenclamide, lithium, vinblastine and colchicine. Renal diseases leading to nephrogenic diabetes insipidus include analgesic nephropathy, relief of urinary obstruction, polycystic disease, medullary cystic disease and interstitial nephritis. Other conditions such as hypocalcaemia, myeloma and amyloidosis may also lead to nephrogenic diabetes insipidus.

30 d e
Parathyroid hormone is produced by the parathyroid glands and calcitonin by the *thyroid*. PTH elevates plasma calcium by increasing osteoclastic activity and decreasing reabsorption of phosphate from the glomerular filtrate. Its actions on bone are dependent upon 1,25-dihydroxycholecalciferol and hence the action of PTH is impaired in the absence of 1,25-DHCC.

31 b
Orthostatic proteinuria is worse in the upright position. Normal people may excrete up to 0.15 g/24 hours; levels above this usually indicate disease. Tubular proteinuria comprises low molecular weight proteins ($\alpha 2$ and β microglobulins) and *glomerular* proteinuria is usually due to albumin. Bence Jones protein will not show on stick testing and is confirmed by Bradshaw's test.

32 a b
Hypomagnesaemia may be secondary to malnutrition, alcoholism, laxative abuse, diuretics, renal tubular acidosis, *hyperthyroidism*, diabetes mellitus and acute pancreatitis amongst other causes. High plasma magnesium may be a result of hypothyroidism, burns, diabetic ketoacidosis, mineralocorticoid deficiency, chronic hypercapnia and rhabdomyolysis. Clinical features of hypomagnesaemia include muscle tremor, tetany, ataxia, anorexia and ECG changes including prolongation of the QT interval and low voltage T waves.

33 Erythropoietin levels are raised in:
- a ovarian carcinoma
- b polycythaemia rubra vera
- c androgen treatment
- d renal failure
- e cardiovascular shunt

34 In patients with ascites:
- a urinary sodium excretion of <5 mmol/day is a recognised finding
- b total body sodium is normal
- c the intravascular volume is reduced
- d if the cause is Budd Chiari syndrome the ascitic fluid will have a high protein content
- e an insidious onset implies a worse prognosis than if the onset is acute

35 Calcitonin:
- a has a steroid structure
- b extracted from salmon is more active in humans than human calcitonin
- c inhibits insulin secretion
- d enhances gastrin secretion
- e deficiency produces major disturbances in skeletal homeostasis

36 Causes of a macrocytosis in the peripheral blood film include:
- a sideroblastic anaemia
- b α thalassaemia
- c red cell aplasia
- d newborn infants
- e chronic respiratory failure

37 The following factors favour iron absorption from the bowel:
- a iron in the ferric form
- b dietary phytate
- c an alkaline environment
- d pregnancy
- e vitamin C

38 Splenomegaly is a feature of:
- a myeloproliferative disorders
- b sarcoidosis
- c iron-deficient anaemia
- d tropical sprue
- e glucose-6-phosphate dehydrogenase deficiency

(Answers overleaf)

33 a c e
Erythropoietin is a glycoprotein. Levels are raised in hypoxia, obesity, haemolysis, haemorrhage, red cell aplasia, renal cysts and carcinoma, cerebellar haemangioblastoma, uterine fibroma and ovarian carcinoma. In renal failure levels are low and in polycythaemia rubra vera levels may be normal or low.

34 a c d e
In cirrhotics sodium retention results in low renal excretion of sodium (<5 mmol/day) and increased total body sodium. Reduction of the intravascular volume also causes the renal tubules to retain sodium compounded by increased aldosterone secretion. Similarly, renin levels are elevated. In cirrhotics the protein content of the ascitic fluid is low (<20 g/l) but in Budd Chiari syndrome it is much higher.

35 b c
Calcitonin is not a steroid hormone but a polypeptide containing 32 amino acids. The whole molecule is required for biological activity. Its actions are roughly opposite to those of parathyroid hormone in that it is responsible for lowering plasma calcium levels by reducing osteoclastic activity and decreasing renal tubular reabsorption of calcium (and sodium, magnesium and potassium). It inhibits secretion of insulin, glucagon and gastrin. Interestingly, in its absence there are only *minor* disturbances in calcium metabolism and homeostasis of the skeleton.

36 a c d e
Sideroblastic anaemia, red cell aplasia and chronic respiratory failure are causes of macrocytosis. Other causes include hypothyroidism, alcoholism, high reticulocyte count, leucoerythroblastic anaemia, pregnancy and aplastic anaemia.

37 d e
Factors favouring absorption of iron from the bowel include anoxia, pregnancy, increased red blood cell production, iron deficiency, low pH, inorganic iron and iron in the *ferrous* form.

38 a b c e
Splenomegaly occurs in lympho- and myeloproliferative disorders. It is also a feature of haemoglobinopathies, haemolytic anaemias, SBE, typhoid fever, tuberculosis, kala-azar, SLE, rheumatoid arthritis, amyloidosis and sarcoidosis.

39 The following conditions are associated with the presence of bilirubin in the urine:
  a   intrahepatic cholestasis
  b   haemolysis
  c   glucuronyl transferase deficiency
  d   hepatocellular damage
  e   physiological jaundice

40 T lymphocytes differ from B lymphocytes in that the former:
  a   have complement receptors on their surface
  b   lack cell surface immunoglobulin
  c   form rosettes with sheep red blood cells
  d   are responsible for humoral immunity
  e   transform into plasma cells

(Answers overleaf)

39 a d
Bilirubin is absent from normal urine and in patients with unconjugated hyperbilirubinaemia (e.g. Gilbert's syndrome, physiological jaundice, haemolysis and glucuronyl transferase deficiency). In patients who are jaundiced and in whom the urine contains bilirubin, hepatocellular disease, cholestasis and conditions such as Rotor/Dubin-Johnston should be considered.

40 b c
T lymphocytes lack complement receptors, Fc receptors and immunoglobulin on their surface. They form rosettes with sheep RBCs but do not transform into plasma cells (this is a function of B lymphocytes). T lymphocytes are responsible for cellular immunity whereas B cells, via immunoglobulin production, are responsible for humoral immunity.

2. Cardiology

1. **Cardiac rupture:**
   a. occurs 2–3 weeks after acute myocardial infarction
   b. is seen more frequently in females than males
   c. is associated with transmural infarction
   d. affects the right and left ventricles in roughly equal frequency
   e. is a known cause of cardiac arrest in sinus rhythm

2. **M-mode is superior to cross-sectional echocardiography for detecting:**
   a. hypertrophy of the left ventricle
   b. tricuspid valve abnormalities
   c. systolic anterior motion in hypertrophic obstructive cardiomyopathy
   d. regional variation in LV function
   e. left atrial enlargement

3. **ECG changes associated with tricyclic antidepressant overdose include:**
   a. short QT interval
   b. bradycardia
   c. prolongation of the PR interval
   d. left axis deviation
   e. increased height of 'U' wave

4. **First degree heart block is a feature of:**
   a. myotonic dystrophy
   b. β blockade
   c. digoxin therapy
   d. subacute bacterial endocarditis
   e. atrial septal defect

(Answers overleaf)

1 b c e
This affects older people and is more common in those who are hypertensive. It tends to occur during the first few days post-infarct. It is also commoner in females, transmural infarcts and left more than right ventricles.

2 a c
In M-mode echocardiography a single ultrasound beam is directed towards the heart. It allows the size and thickness of intracardiac structures to be measured. Cross-sectional echocardiography uses multiple beams and its images are easier to interpret. M-mode is useful in detecting LVH, mitral valve vibrations in aortic regurgitation, LV filling rate in mitral stenosis and systolic anterior motion seen in HOCM. Cross-sectional echocardiography is better for measuring mitral and aortic valve areas, abnormalities of the pulmonary and tricuspid valves and regional variations in LV function.

3 c e
Tricyclic antidepressants produce effects on the ECG similar to those seen with quinidine treatment, i.e. low voltage T waves, ST depression, prolonged QT interval and wide P waves.

4 a b c d e
First degree heart block is caused by delayed conduction through the conducting system. The PR interval is prolonged (>0.20 sec). All impulses reach the ventricles. It may occasionally be a feature of normal people and also occurs in rheumatic fever but more commonly in digoxin toxicity.

CARDIOLOGY

5 Prolongation of the QT interval may be seen in:
 a patients with increased intracranial pressure
 b patients receiving phenothiazines
 c hypothermia
 d hypercalcaemia
 e thyrotoxicosis

6 Reversed splitting of the second heart sound occurs in:
 a aortic stenosis
 b patent ductus arteriosus
 c atrial septal defect
 d left bundle branch block
 e anomalous pulmonary venous drainage

7 A venous hum in the neck:
 a is usually louder in systole
 b is maximal with the head turned away
 c increases during expiration
 d is best heard with the patient lying flat
 e is abolished by finger pressure over the internal jugular vein

8 The following are true of the Wolff-Parkinson-White syndrome:
 a it occurs most frequently in males
 b a QRS complex of >0.1 sec is diagnostic
 c the T wave is upright in lead aVL
 d the first heart sound is loud
 e life expectancy is reduced

9 A short PR interval on the ECG occurs in:
 a Duchenne muscular dystrophy
 b Lown-Ganong-Levine syndrome
 c hypertrophic obstructive cardiomyopathy
 d hypokalaemia
 e digoxin toxicity

10 Causes of a dominant R wave in lead V1 include:
 a pulmonary hypertension
 b Wolff-Parkinson-White syndrome type B
 c dextrocardia
 d amyloidosis
 e hypertrophic obstructive cardiomyopathy

11 A soft first heart sound is a feature of:
 a mitral incompetence
 b tachycardia
 c first degree heart block
 d Wolff-Parkinson-White syndrome
 e pericardial effusion

(Answers overleaf)

5 a b c
The QT interval is normally 0.33–0.43 sec. It becomes longer in bradycardia and shorter with tachycardia. Other causes of prolongation include: myocardial infarction, quinidine, procainamide, amiodarone and hypothermia.

6 a b d
The second sound is normally split in inspiration (A_2P_2) but when the sound is split in expiration and has the P_2A_2 configuration this should raise suspicions about the possibility of left bundle branch block, severe aortic stenosis, LVF, patent ductus arteriosus or HOCM.

7 b e
A venous hum is a blowing continuous murmur, is heard maximally at the base of the heart and diminishes with the child lying flat.

8 a d e
Wolff-Parkinson-White is one of the pre-excitation syndromes and affects 1% of the population. It is due to an accessory conduction pathway which bypasses the AV node leading to a short PR interval and prolongation of the QRS complex. Re-entry circuits may produce SVT. The condition is associated with mitral valve prolapse, hypertrophic obstructive cardiomyopathy, Ebstein's anomaly, male gender and may be familial.

9 a b c
The normal PR interval is 0.12–0.20 sec. A short PR interval is seen in AV nodal rhythm, hypertrophic obstructive cardiomyopathy (HOCM), Duchenne muscular dystrophy and Wolff-Parkinson-White syndrome. A long PR interval is seen in digoxin toxicity, hypo- and hyperkalaemia as well as first degree heart block.

10 a c e
Causes of a dominant R wave in lead V1 include: Wolff-Parkinson-White syndrome type A, true posterior myocardial infarct, pulmonary hypertension, ASD, right bundle branch block, HOCM and dextrocardia.

11 a c e
The first heart sound represents the closure of the mitral and tricuspid valves once the ventricular pressure exceeds that in the atria. A soft first heart sound is heard in left ventricular failure, mitral regurgitation, first degree heart block, emphysema and pericardial effusion. A loud first heart sound occurs in conditions associated with a hyperdynamic circulation such as thyrotoxicosis, WPW syndrome and also mitral stenosis.

CARDIOLOGY

12 Contraindications to exercise testing include:
a left bundle branch block
b patients with presumptive exercise-induced arrhythmias
c patients started on digoxin in the previous 7 days
d severe aortic stenosis
e prolonged ischaemic chest pain within the past 24 hours

13 Diagnostic criteria for right ventricular hypertrophy include:
a R wave in aVL >13 mm
b T inversion in leads facing the left ventricle
c QRS duration <0.12 sec
d dominant R wave in lead V1
e frontal QRS plane more positive than +90°

14 The following are associated with a low HDL:cholesterol ratio:
a androgens
b moderate alcohol
c regular exercise
d β blockers
e dietary sugar

15 The following findings in a patient support the diagnosis of constrictive pericarditis:
a blood pressure which falls on expiration
b JVP which rises on inspiration
c pulse volume which decreases with inspiration
d slow 'y' descent in the JVP
e splenomegaly

16 The following drugs lower the blood pressure by reducing afterload predominantly:
a nitrates
b phentolamine
c nifedipine
d morphine
e frusemide

17 Primary pulmonary hypertension is associated with:
a pregnancy
b scleroderma
c Hurler's syndrome
d fourth heart sound
e normal pulmonary artery wedge pressure

(Answers overleaf)

12 a c d e
Patients should not undergo exercise testing if they have recently been started on digoxin, have documented recurrent ventricular tachyarrhythmias, have known aortic stenosis or have had a recent episode of prolonged chest pain.

13 c d e
Criteria for RVH are: dominant R in V1, absence of anterolateral infarction, QRS <0.12 sec and frontal QRS more positive than +90°.
a and **b** are criteria for LVH.

14 a d e
Increased HDL:cholesterol ratios may be seen in patients who are F > M, take regular exercise and moderate alcohol and are of higher educational status.

15 b c e
Constrictive pericarditis may be secondary to tuberculous pericarditis. The blood pressure rises with expiration, the JVP rises with inspiration (cf normal), ascites may be present as might an S_3 (or pericardial knock). Ventricular filling will be reduced.

16 b c
Afterload reducers include: hydralazine, phentolamine, nifedipine and captopril. Preload reducers are: morphine, frusemide and nitrates. Those which have combined pre- and afterload effects are: nitroprusside and prazosin.

17 a b d e
This is a diagnosis of exclusion and tends to affect young females. It is associated with a number of conditions including scleroderma, Raynaud's and SLE. Signs include a low cardiac output, prominent 'a' waves in the JVP, S_4 and parasternal heave.

CARDIOLOGY

18 A patient who has recently sustained a myocardial infarct might be considered as having polyarteritis nodosa if the following were found:
  a focal glomerulonephritis
  b monocytosis on peripheral blood film
  c peripheral neuropathy
  d pancreatitis
  e fibrosing alveolitis

19 In a child with congenital heart disease, prominent pulmonary vasculature on CXR would support a diagnosis of:
  a Eisenmenger's syndrome
  b patent ductus arteriosus
  c primary pulmonary hypertension
  d Fallot's tetralogy
  e ventricular septal defect

20 Anti-arrhythmic agents which act predominantly on ventricular tissues include:
  a mexiletine
  b β blockers
  c digoxin
  d disopyramide
  e lignocaine

21 The following are true of left atrial myxoma:
  a it is commoner in males
  b finger clubbing is a feature
  c histology is always benign
  d pulmonary hypertension is a complication
  e the ECG may be diagnostic

22 A fourth heart sound occurs in:
  a atrial fibrillation
  b heart block
  c hypertrophic obstructive cardiomyopathy
  d heart failure
  e hypertension

23 The following signs, if found in a pregnant woman, warrant further investigation:
  a third heart sound
  b prominent 'a' wave in the JVP
  c an early diastolic murmur
  d ankle oedema
  e systemic hypertension

(Answers overleaf)

18 a c d
Polyarteritis nodosa affects older men > women and is associated with focal glomerulonephritis, peripheral neuropathy, asthma and myocardial infarction. Findings are: raised white blood cell count (neutrophils, eosinophilia) and positive hepatitis B serology.

19 b e
Those conditions with plethoric lung fields include: ASD, VSD, PDA and left to right shunts. Diseases associated with decreased pulmonary vasculature are: pulmonary stenosis. Fallot's tetralogy and pulmonary atresia.

20 a e
β blockers and digoxin act on the AV node; disopyramide produces effects on atrial tissue, accessory pathways and ventricular tissue.

21 b c d
Left atrial myxoma is not strictly an accurate term since this tumour can originate in the right atrium (less commonly). It may mimic mitral stenosis and produces constitutional symptoms such as anaemia, clubbing, pyrexia and malaise. The ESR is raised but the CXR and ECG may not be helpful. The histology is benign and recurrence post-excision can occur.

22 b c d e
A fourth heart sound is due to atrial contraction and occurs before S_1. No S_4 is heard in atrial fibrillation.

23 c e
In pregnancy ankle oedema as well as prominent 'a' and 'v' waves in the JVP are not uncommon. The apex may be hyperdynamic and a systolic flow murmur may be heard. Cyanosis, persistent hypertension, generalised oedema and the presence of a diastolic murmur warrants further investigation.

CARDIOLOGY

24 Right axis deviation may be due to:
  a left anterior hemiblock
  b chronic obstructive airways disease
  c myotonic dystrophy
  d Wolff-Parkinson-White syndrome
  e primum atrial septal defect

25 ECG characteristics of ventricular tachycardia which help differentiate it from supraventricular tachycardia include:
  a normal QRS axis
  b ventricular rate >170/minute
  c mono- or biphasic QRS
  d fusion beats
  e QRS <0.14 sec

26 The following are causes of right bundle branch block:
  a congenital
  b ischaemic heart disease
  c secundum atrial septal defect
  d aortic stenosis
  e fibrosis of conducting tissue

27 The following statements about the jugular venous pressure (JVP) are true:
  a giant 'a' waves are seen in tricuspid incompetence
  b 'a' waves are absent in ventricular tachycardia
  c the 'y' descent is absent in nodal rhythm
  d 'v' waves reflect atrial relaxation
  e the JVP normally rises with inspiration

28 Features consistent with a diagnosis of restrictive cardiomyopathy include:
  a third heart sound
  b variable atheroma
  c normal-sized left ventricle
  d double apical impulse
  e myocardial fibre disarray

29 Major criteria used in the diagnosis of rheumatic fever include:
  a erythema multiforme
  b arthralgia
  c prolonged PR interval on ECG
  d chorea
  e subcutaneous nodules

(Answers overleaf)

24 none
All those listed are causes of left axis deviation. Right axis deviation may be due to cor pulmonale, pulmonary stenosis, Fallot's tetralogy, right bundle branch block, pulmonary embolism and anterolateral myocardial infarction.

25 c d
In VT the rate is often <170/ minute, QRS is >0.14 sec, LAD is present as are fusion beats. Other signs include cannon waves in the JVP, variable S_1 and beat-to-beat variation in blood pressure.

26 a b c e
RBBB may be normal but is sometimes found in pulmonary hypertension and pulmonary embolism. LBBB is almost always abnormal and is seen in ischaemic heart disease, aortic stenosis and cardiomyopathy.

27 b
Giant 'a' waves are seen in pulmonary hypertension, pulmonary stenosis and tricuspid stenosis. The normal 'y' descent is absent in tamponade and superior vena cava obstruction. The 'v' wave is due to venous filling of the atria and the JVP normally drops on inspiration.

28 a c
This is the least common disease of heart muscle and may be caused by a variety of conditions including: amyloid, eosinophilic heart disease (Löffler's eosinophilia), neoplastic infiltration, Fabry's disease, carcinoid and African cardiomyopathy. Ventricular compliance is reduced. Both S_3 and S_4 occur and there may be a pansystolic murmur in the mitral or tricuspid areas. Venous pressure is increased with deep 'x' and 'y' descent. Using echocardiography the cavities may be seen to be normal in size.

29 d e
Major criteria are: carditis, polyarthritis, chorea, erythema marginatum (not itchy), subcutaneous nodules and evidence of streptococcal infection
Minor criteria are: fever, arthralgia, previous rheumatic fever, raised ESR and prolonged PR interval.
To make the diagnosis:

Two major criteria are needed *or* one major + two minor.

30 Causes of cyanotic congenital heart disease include:
- a patent ductus arteriosus
- b pulmonary stenosis
- c primum atrial septal defect
- d tricuspid atresia
- e coarctation of the aorta

(Answer overleaf)

30 d
The causes of cyanotic congenital heart disease include Fallot's tetralogy, transposition of the great vessels, tricuspid atresia and Eisenmenger's syndrome.

3. Dermatology

1. **Café au lait spots occur in the following:**
   a. thyrotoxicosis
   b. phaeochromocytoma
   c. Whipple's disease
   d. sarcoidosis
   e. subacute bacterial endocarditis

2. **In a patient suffering from a bullous skin disease, pemphigus is more likely than pemphigoid if:**
   a. the patient has myasthenia gravis
   b. the bullae are subepidermal
   c. the lesions fail to demonstrate Nikolsky's sign
   d. lesions are more prominent on the arms and thighs
   e. the condition has an insidious onset

3. **Erythema multiforme:**
   a. is commoner in females
   b. is associated with arthralgia
   c. is commonly associated with leukaemia
   d. occurs as a consequence of viral infection
   e. seldom affects the face

4. **Fixed drug eruptions occur with the following:**
   a. barbiturates
   b. gold
   c. phenylbutazone
   d. captopril
   e. penicillin

5. **The following conditions are associated with leg ulceration:**
   a. polyarteritis nodosa
   b. hypothyroidism
   c. spinal cord lesions
   d. syphilis
   e. hereditary spherocytosis

(Answers overleaf)

1 a b e
Café au lait spots represent macular hyperpigmentation and occur in multiple neurofibromatosis, subacute bacterial endocarditis, phaeochromocytoma, thyrotoxicosis and Albright's disease.

2 a e
Both are blistering conditions. Pemphigus (F>M, commoner in Jews) tends to be chronic, progressive and fatal. Lesions demonstrate Nikolsky's sign and are associated with autoimmune conditions. Pemphigoid is commoner than pemphigus, is chronic but benign, has IgG on the basement membrane and may be associated with underlying malignancy. The blister in pemphigus is *intra*-epidermal and in pemphigoid is *sub*epidermal.

3 a b d
Erythema multiforme affects the hands and feet predominantly and blisters are subepidermal. It may be idiopathic or secondary to drugs (sulphonamides, penicillins and phenobarbitone), or viral, bacterial and *Mycoplasma* infections.

4 a b c d e
These are common and often take the form of a toxic erythematous rash. However, morbilliform, psoriasiform and pemphigus-like rashes occur. Drugs involved include sulphonamides, penicillins, phenylbutazone, salicylates, phenothiazines and tetracyclines.

5 a c d e
Leg ulcers may be due to venous stasis (common), infection (gas gangrene, Buruli ulcer, tuberculosis, leprosy, syphilis and yaws), trauma, bites, metabolic disease (diabetes mellitus), vasculitis, neoplasia (epithelioma, Kaposi's sarcoma and melanoma), ischaemia, arterial disease (hypertension, temporal arteritis), thrombosis, coagulopathies and neuropathies.

DERMATOLOGY

6 Vitiligo is associated with:
  a hyperthyroidism
  b morphoea
  c polyarteritis nodosa
  d halo naevus
  e malignant melanoma

7 Photosensitive eruptions are caused by:
  a penicillins
  b nalidixic acid
  c amiodarone
  d aminophylline
  e griseofulvin

8 The following are associated with blue nails:
  a chloroquine treatment
  b Pseudomonas infection
  c Wilson's disease
  d argyria
  e tetracycline treatment

9 Drugs known to cause alopecia include:
  a colchicine
  b metronidazole
  c carbimazole
  d methyldopa
  e ethionamide

10 The following are premalignant:
  a basal cell papilloma
  b actinic keratosis
  c kerato-acanthoma
  d histiocytoma
  e pyogenic granuloma

(Answers overleaf)

6 a b d
Vitiligo represents an area of cutaneous depigmentation. Associations include autoimmune conditions such as pernicious anaemia, Addison's disease, thyroid disease, hypoparathyroidism and alopecia areata.

7 b c e
There are numerous causes of photosensitivity including SLE, xeroderma pigmentosum and porphyria. Drugs causing photosensitive rashes include phenothiazines, tetracyclines, chlorpropamide, nalidixic acid, griseofulvin and tar products.

8 a c d
Nails may change colour in a variety of conditions, e.g. yellow nails (yellow nail syndrome) associated with pleural effusions and lymphoedema; white nails and liver disease/hypoalbuminaemia.

9 a c e
Alopecia may be idiopathic or acquired. Drugs which cause it include heparin, cyclophosphamide and methotrexate.

10 b
The incidence of basal cell papilloma increases with advancing age. Biopsy may be necessary to exclude malignancy. Actinic keratoses are hyperpigmented and develop on exposed areas. They may transform into squamous cell carcinoma.

4. Endocrinology

1. **Recognised causes of gynaecomastia include:**
   a. pituitary failure
   b. coeliac disease
   c. chronic renal failure
   d. hyperthyroidism
   e. bronchial carcinoma

2. **Unilateral exophthalmos is seen in:**
   a. myasthenia gravis
   b. rhinocerebral mucormycosis
   c. Wegener's granulomatosis
   d. Grave's disease
   e. meningioma

3. **Conditions predisposing to recurrent hypoglycaemia include:**
   a. acromegaly
   b. hypothyroidism
   c. renal failure
   d. autonomic neuropathy
   e. diabetes insipidus

4. **The following oral hypoglycaemic drugs are eliminated predominantly by hepatic metabolism:**
   a. chlorpropamide
   b. glibenclamide
   c. tolbutamide
   d. metformin
   e. glipizide

5. **Biochemical findings which would support a diagnosis of inappropriate antidiuretic hormone secretion include:**
   a. urine of low specific gravity
   b. increased urine osmolality
   c. serum Na^+ of 115 mmol/l
   d. low serum osmolality
   e. hyperkalaemia

(Answers overleaf)

1 a c d e
Gynaecomastia is enlargement of the male breast due to an increase in breast tissue. Galactorrhoea may be due to hyperprolactinaemia but there is no association between hyperprolactinaemia and gynaecomastia. Various tumours (carcinoma of bronchus, breast and liver) have been reported to cause gynaecomastia and are associated with high circulating levels of chorionic gonadotrophin and leutenising hormone.

2 b c d e
Unilateral exophthalmos may be caused by dysthyroidism, orbital inflammation, granulomas and cysts. Pulsating exophthalmos is caused by caroticocavernous fistula. Bilateral eye disease is more characteristic of thyroid disease but can also be a developmental abnormality.

3 b c d
Hypoglycaemia has numerous causes including gastric surgery, fructose intolerance, insulinoma, fibrosarcoma, alcohol abuse, nesidioblastoma (rare). Von Gierke's disease and galactosaemia.

4 b c e
Oral hypoglycaemic drugs fall into two categories: (1) sulphonylureas and (2) biguanides. The sulphonylureas such as tolbutamide, chlorpropamide and glibenclamide act by augmenting endogenous insulin secretion. All may lead to hypoglycaemia. The biguanides (metformin; phenformin is no longer used) act by decreasing gluconeogenesis and increase the peripheral utilisation of glucose. This group should not be used in patients with renal failure because of the risk of lactic acidosis.

5 b c d
SIADH leads to hyponatraemia and the urine will be inappropriately concentrated. The patient will be in approximate sodium balance. The syndrome may be due to lung cancer, head injury, pneumonia, hypothyroidism or porphyria.

ENDOCRINOLOGY

6 In thyroid carcinoma:
   a follicular carcinoma is associated with other endocrine abnormalities
   b papillary carcinoma carries a relatively good prognosis
   c medullary carcinoma may secrete ACTH
   d regression of papillary carcinoma with thyroxine is recognised
   e thyroid carcinoma is often associated with hyperthyroidism

7 Aldosterone:
   a secretion is dependent upon ACTH
   b is stimulated by an increase in circulating renin levels
   c if produced by tumour of the adrenal cortex may raise the serum pH
   d secretion is increased in oedematous states
   e in excess leads to impaired glucose tolerance

8 The following conditions are associated with glucose intolerance:
   a coeliac disease
   b Huntington's chorea
   c retinitis pigmentosa
   d Down's syndrome
   e treatment with diazoxide

9 Growth hormone deficiency is found in:
   a dermatomyositis
   b pygmies
   c hypothyroidism
   d Marfan's syndrome
   e pineal tumour

10 Features of pseudohypoparathyroidism include:
   a subnormal levels of parathyroid hormone (PTH)
   b increased renal excretion of cAMP on administration of PTH
   c short metatarsals
   d an association with hypothyroidism
   e all target tissues resistant to PTH

11 Hypopituitarism occurs in:
   a syphilis
   b neurofibromatosis
   c emotional deprivation
   d cranial arteritis
   e basal skull fracture

(Answers overleaf)

6 **b c d**
Anaplastic and medullary carcinoma occur in older patients. Medullary tumours may secrete calcitonin which serves as a marker in screening relatives. Prognosis is poor. Papillary tumours affect younger people and may present as lateral aberrant thyroid. Treatment is with thyroxine and the prognosis is good. Thyroid cancer is rarely associated with hyperthyroidism.

7 **b c d e**
Aldosterone is involved in the control of Na^+ and K^+ homeostasis. Secretion is controlled by, amongst other factors, hypotension and reduced circulating blood volume. When deficient, K^+ retention and Na^+ loss occurs. Its effects are mainly exerted on the distal tubule and collecting ducts of the kidney.

8 **a b c d e**
A 'lag storage' glucose tolerance curve may be seen in chronic liver disease, thyrotoxicosis and the dumping syndrome. A 'flat' GTT occurs in malabsorption and Addison's disease. The curve may be frankly diabetic in patients on corticosteroids.

9 **b c e**
Growth hormone has anti-insulin properties. Deficiency in adults has no serious effects but in children leads to dwarfism. In excess it may be produced by adenomas of the pituitary gland and results in acromegaly (adults) and gigantism (children). Growth hormone excess may be assessed by (1) basal GH level and (2) oral glucose tolerance test.

10 **c d**
This is an uncommon inborn error of metabolism and reflects the decreased response of the kidney and bone to parathyroid hormone (PTH). Plasma calcium falls and PTH levels rise. The effect of 1α-cholecalciferol hydroxylase is impaired.

11 **a b c d e**
Hypopituitarism may be caused by a variety of conditions including granulomas, tumour (primary or secondary deposits); inflammatory conditions such as cranial arteritis, post-surgery/radiotherapy, head injury, infection (syphilis and meningitis) and pituitary apoplexy. The clinical picture depends on the hormone deficiency. The most common cause is a prolactinoma in adults.

12 Glucagon:
a is a polypeptide containing 29 amino acids
b decreases cAMP production
c is secreted in response to a protein meal
d is produced from pro-glucagon
e release is stimulated by somatostatin

13 Concerning congenital adrenal hyperplasia:
a in 21-hydroxylase deficiency there is decreased 17-hydroxyprogesterone
b 21-hydroxylase deficiency leads to a salt-losing state
c treatment is aimed at suppressing ACTH and hence androgen production
d 17-hydroxylase deficiency is the commonest form
e 21-hydroxylase deficiency is inherited in an autosomal recessive manner

14 The following findings are compatible with a diagnosis of Addison's disease:
a hypoglycaemia
b hypokalaemia
c hypernatraemia
d hypercalcaemia
e elevated blood urea

15 Acromegaly is commonly associated with:
a cardiomyopathy
b headache
c osteoporosis
d auditory defects
e decreased libido

16 The following are features of Cushing's disease rather than ectopic adrenocorticotrophic hormone (ACTH) secretion secondary to oat cell carcinoma of the bronchus:
a weight loss
b response to dexamethasone
c oedema is rare
d response to metyrapone
e diabetic glucose tolerance test

(Answers overleaf)

12 a c d
Glucagon is a single chain polypeptide synthesised by the α cells of the pancreas, gastric fundus and duodenum and is stimulated by hypoglycaemia, starvation, oral arginine and stress. Its effects are: stimulated glycogenolysis, stimulated gluconeogenesis and prevention of hepatic glycogen synthesis.

13 b c e
This is a group of inherited disorders and may be 21-, 17- or 11-hydroxylase deficiency. Cortisol production is impaired and intermediate metabolites accumulate. 21-hydroxylase deficiency is the commonest and, in this, 17-hydroxprogesterone accumulates. Since this is an androgen precursor males show accelerated sexual development and females are virilised.

14 a d e
Addison's disease (chronic hypo-adrenalism) may be primary or secondary. Primary causes include autoimmune disease and secondary causes may be due to tumour infiltration or granulomatous disease. Patients complain of tiredness, gastrointestinal complaints, pigmentation and may be found to have hypoglycaemia, raised urea, hyponatraemia and hyperkalaemia. Tests for Addison's disease include: short synacthen test and serum ACTH measurements.

15 b c
Most cases are due to acidophil adenoma of the pituitary. Bone and soft tissue increase in bulk, facial appearances may alter with the development of prognathism, increased size of frontal and other sinuses, visual field defects, cardiomegaly and hypertension. Headache and osteoporosis are common. Cardiomyopathy, auditory defects and decreased libido, although they occur, are not the *common* manifestations

16 c d
Cushing's syndrome may be due to (1) Cushing's disease which is pituitary-dependent adrenal hyperplasia, (2) adrenal tumours and (3) ectopic ACTH secretion or exogenous hormone administration. ACTH levels are very high in ectopic ACTH secretion and fail to suppress with dexamethasone because secretion of ACTH by the pituitary is already suppressed by high circulating levels and dexamethasone, therefore, has no effect. Weight loss is commoner in Cushing's syndrome due to bronchial carcinoma than in pituitary-dependent Cushing's disease. In the metyrapone test there is an increase in urinary 17-oxogenic steroids in pituitary-dependent Cushing's disease but *no* rise is seen in non-pituitary-dependent forms of Cushing's syndrome. The most useful investigations are: 9 a.m. and midnight cortisols, dexamethasone suppression test, 24-hour urinary free cortisol and insulin stress test.

ENDOCRINOLOGY

17 **Dopamine agonists include:**
   a apomorphine
   b butyrophenones
   c metoclopramide
   d bromocriptine
   e reserpine

18 **Ovarian tumours which secrete androgens include:**
   a struma ovarii
   b arrhenoblastoma
   c granulosa cell tumour
   d hilar cell tumour
   e thecoma

19 **Raised thyroid binding globulin is found in:**
   a acute porphyria
   b acromegaly
   c patients taking the oral contraceptive pill
   d prolonged phenothiazine treatment
   e severe illness

20 **The following statements about phaeochromocytoma are true:**
   a tumours originating in bladder are recognised
   b there is an association with papillary thyroid carcinoma
   c dopamine may be secreted by malignant tumours
   d headache is primarily an alpha adrenergic effect
   e hypertension is sustained in only a minority of cases

(Answers overleaf)

17 a d
Dopamine, L-dopa, apomorphine and bromocriptine are dopamine *agonists*. Phenothiazines, butyrophenones and metoclopramide are dopamine *antagonists*. Reserpine is a dopamine-depleting agent.

18 b d
Arrhenoblastoma, like hilar cell tumours, secrete androgens. Granulosa cell tumours and thecomas secrete oestrogens. Struma ovarii tumours secrete thyroxine.

19 a c d
TBG is an α-globulin to which almost all T4 and T3 is bound. A rise in TBG results in a rise in bound T4 and T4 binding sites which are unoccupied. Causes include: newborn babies, oral contraceptive and porphyria. Decreased TBG is seen in patients on androgens, nephrotic syndrome and severe illness.

20 a c d
Phaeochromocytoma is a tumour of the adrenal medulla and is associated with MEA II (medullary thyroid carcinoma, parathyroid adenoma/carcinoma and phaeochromocytoma). It may originate in other sites such as the bladder and these are tumours of adults. The histology is usually benign. Clinical features include paroxysmal hypertension, sweating, anxiety, flushing. Hyperglycaemia and glycosuria are associated.

5. Gastroenterology

1. **The following statements concerning achalasia are true:**
   a. achalasia affects only the lower third of the oesophagus
   b. barium swallow examination may be normal
   c. inhalation of octyl nitrite aids the differentiation between achalasia and carcinoma
   d. inheritance is autosomal dominant with variable penetrance
   e. anticholinergic drugs reduce the force of sphincter contraction

2. **Concerning hepatocellular carcinoma:**
   a. it is found in high frequency amongst the Bantu tribe
   b. *Aspergillus flavus* toxin is a predisposing cause
   c. specific HLA antigens have been shown to correlate with development of the tumour
   d. this tumour has been shown to follow massive immunosuppression in renal transplant patients
   e. primary liver cancer is a frequent cause of death in patients with haemochromatosis

3. **The following are causes of acute pancreatitis:**
   a. hypercalcaemia
   b. hyperthermia
   c. corticosteroids
   d. systemic lupus erythematosus
   e. thrombotic thrombocytopenic purpura

4. **In the Zollinger-Ellison syndrome (gastrinoma):**
   a. there is an association with MEA type II
   b. the finding of hypergastrinaemia confirms the diagnosis
   c. the pathology lies in the beta cells of the pancreas
   d. diarrhoea is an early symptom
   e. CAT scanning is useful in diagnosis in most cases

(Answers overleaf)

1 b c e
Achalasia is due to degeneration of myenteric ganglion cells of the whole oesophagus. Manometry shows non-peristaltic contraction and increased intra-oesophageal pressure associated with progressive atony and dilatation. Dysphagia may be intermittent and aspiration is a risk. There is an increased incidence of oesophageal carcinoma in patients with achalasia. Barium swallow may be normal or show the distal oesophagus terminating in a 'beak'. Inhalation of octyl nitrite relaxes the smooth muscle transiently and may aid in the differentiation between achalasia and carcinoma.

2 a b d e
Hepatocellular carcinoma has been linked to several factors including cirrhosis, alcohol, haemochromatosis, aflatoxin (*A. flavus*) and hepatitis B. It is common amongst the Bantu tribe who use iron cooking pots. There has been no good evidence of genetic or HLA association. Histology shows tumour cells in blood spaces and the cells are smaller than normal liver cells with granular cytoplasm.

3 a c d e
Common causes of acute pancreatitis are: alcohol abuse, gallstones and trauma. Among the less common causes are sulphasalazine, steroids, thiazides, mumps, hyperparathyroidism, SLE and viral hepatitis. Complications include pseudocyst formation, pancreatic abscess, hyperglycaemia, hypocalcaemia and hypoalbuminaemia.

4 d
Zollinger-Ellison syndrome is a condition of the pancreatic non-beta islet cells leading to hypergastrinaemia and recurrent duodenal ulceration. Diagnosis is by raised fasting gastrin levels. It is associated with MEA I (hyperparathyroidism, pituitary adenoma). High gastrin levels are not diagnostic and may be found in other conditions such as patients who have not fasted, achlorhydria and chronic renal failure. CAT scanning is not useful in picking up small tumours.

GASTROENTEROLOGY

5 The following statements regarding primary biliary cirrhosis (PBC) are true:
   a it is commoner in males
   b cholangiography is usually normal
   c there is an association between PBC and Hashimoto's thyroiditis
   d corticosteroids are useful in providing symptomatic relief
   e copper retention by the liver may reach the levels found in Wilson's disease

6 The following are common causes of hepatic granulomata:
   a talcum
   b tuberculosis
   c Q fever
   d sarcoidosis
   e schistosomiasis

7 Regarding dissolution of gall stones by medical treatment:
   a obesity is a relative contra-indication
   b radiolucent stones dissolve less easily than those which are radio-opaque
   c the stone diameter should be less than 1 cm
   d a functioning gallbladder should be seen on cholecystography
   e there is less diarrhoea with ursodeoxycholic acid than with chenodeoxycholic acid

8 The following dietary agents are allowed in a gluten-free diet:
   a corn
   b rye
   c malt
   d rice
   e soya

9 In cases of antibiotic-induced pseudomembranous colitis the following agents are frequent causes:
   a clindamycin
   b ampicillin
   c griseofulvin
   d vancomycin
   e metronidazole

10 Crohn's disease is associated with:
    a ureteric obstruction
    b thrombo-embolism
    c hirsutism
    d growth retardation
    e osteopenia

(Answers overleaf)

5 **b c e**
PBC is a condition of middle-aged females and is associated with xanthelasmata, pruritus, jaundice and hepatosplenomegaly. Antimitochondrial antibodies are present in 95% of cases and IgM is elevated. Antismooth muscle antibodies may also be present. Liver biopsy shows granulomata. PBC is associated with Sjögren's syndrome, renal tubular acidosis (RTA), pernicious anaemia and thyrotoxicosis. Treatment is with azathioprine and penicillamine. Pruritus may be improved with cholestyramine.

6 **b d e**
Talcum and Q-fever are *rare* causes of hepatic granulomata. The commoner ones are tuberculosis, schistosomiasis and sarcoidosis.

7 **a c d e**
Radiolucent stones are easier to dissolve. A functioning gallbladder is required and patient compliance is paramount. Treatment tends to be prolonged but is useful in selected cases and where surgery cannot be used, e.g. in heart or lung disease.

8 **a d e**
Coeliac disease is believed to be due to gluten/gluten breakdown product sensitivity. Small bowel shows blunted and flattened mucosa with loss of villi. HLA associations are HLA B8 and DW3. Treatment is with gluten-free diet and this excludes oats, rye, barley, malt and wheat. Rice, soya and corn are allowed.

9 **a b**
Antibiotics implicated include lincomycin, ampicillin, clindamycin, erythromycin, cotrimoxazole and metronidazole. It is due to the enterotoxin of *Clostridium difficile*. Treatment consists of oral vancomycin.

10 **a b d e**
Crohn's disease may cause hydronephrosis and oxalate stones. Other complications include fistula formation, bowel obstruction, malabsorption, finger clubbing, aphthous ulceration, uveitis, pericholangitis and gallstone formation.

GASTROENTEROLOGY

11 Presence of HBsAg (hepatitis B surface antigen) is associated with:
  a haemophilia
  b glue sniffing
  c male homosexuals
  d temporal arteritis
  e narcotic addiction

12 In amoebic liver abscess:
  a the right and left lobes are affected in roughly equal frequency
  b liver function tests are usually abnormal
  c a large liquefied space is often detected in the affected lobe
  d culture of the organism is relatively easy if the contents of the abscess are aspirated
  e drainage of the abscess is mandatory

13 In a patient with inflammatory bowel disease a diagnosis of Crohn's is more likely than ulcerative colitis if the following are found:
  a the patient is a smoker
  b transmural involvement
  c loss of goblet cells
  d aphthous oral ulceration
  e non-caseating granulomata

14 Familial unconjugated hyperbilirubinaemia:
  a affects about 5% of the population
  b is commoner in fast acetylators
  c is precipitated by stress
  d may be treated prophylactically by phenytoin
  e leads to a reduction in life expectancy

15 Chronic active hepatitis is associated with:
  a methyldopa
  b aspirin
  c nonA-nonB hepatitis
  d primary biliary cirrhosis
  e oxyphenacetin

16 Features consistent with a diagnosis of Wilson's disease (hepatolenticular degeneration) include:
  a presentation usually in adulthood
  b reduced urinary copper
  c increased hepatic copper
  d dysarthria
  e increased serum uric acid

(Answers overleaf)

11 a c e
There is an increased incidence of HBsAg in haemophiliacs, patients on haemodialysis, polyarteritis nodosa, male homosexuals and intravenous drug abusers.

12 c
This may present as a pyrexia of unknown origin. The right lobe is affected more commonly than the left. Needle aspiration may produce so-called 'anchovy sauce' but culture of *Entamoeba histolytica* is often difficult. Treatment is with metronidazole and large cavities should be aspirated.

13 a b e
Aphthous ulceration is a feature of both conditions and loss of goblet cells is a feature of ulcerative colitis. Other histological features of Crohn's disease include non-caseating granulomata, focal inflammation and infiltration with lymphocytes, macrophages and histiocytes. In ulcerative colitis there are crypt abscesses, decreased numbers of crypts and infiltration with polymorphs, lymphocytes, eosinophils and plasma cells. Interestingly, most patients with ulcerative colitis are non-smokers and, although hardly a reliable guide, a patient who smokes is more likely to have Crohn's disease.

14 a c
Gilbert's disease is due to a mild deficiency of UDP glucuronyl transferase and causes mild unconjugated hyperbilirubinaemia. The condition affects about 5% of the population. It is exacerbated by intercurrent illness, stress, fasting and alcohol. Phenobarbitone may be used as prophylaxis against attacks due to its enzyme-inducing properties. Liver function, histology and life expectancy are normal.

15 a c d e
Chronic active hepatitis may be caused by hepatitis B, nonA-nonB hepatitis, isoniazid, methyldopa, nitrofurantoin, Wilson's disease, ulcerative colitis and α-1 antitrypsin deficiency. The condition affects people between 25 and 50 years of age. There is cirrhosis and piecemeal necrosis. Presentation may be as non-resolving hepatitis, portal hypertension, relapsing jaundice, hirsutism, ascites and bleeding varices.

16 c d e
Wilson's disease is caused by a defect in caeruloplasmin and copper is deposited in the liver and brain. Kayser-Fleischer rings may be present, the serum copper is low and urinary copper is elevated. Liver biopsy shows increased deposition of copper. Complications include RTA, chondrocalcinosis, pigmentation and blue nails.

GASTROENTEROLOGY

17 The following drugs produce a predominantly cholestatic jaundice:
- a phenacetin
- b testosterone
- c methyldopa
- d erythromycin
- e carbimazole

18 The following are features of carcinoid tumours:
- a the carcinoid syndrome occurs in about 50% of carcinoid tumours
- b the tumour may originate in the bronchus
- c methysergide treatment helps flushing mainly
- d the carcinoid syndrome is not produced by colorectal tumours
- e a dermatosis similar to pellagra is recognised

19 Carcinoma of the stomach has an increased frequency in:
- a people of blood group B
- b patients who have had gastric surgery
- c pernicious anaemia
- d primary hypogammaglobulinaemia
- e North America

20 The following statements regarding the Norwalk virus are correct:
- a it affects patients of all ages
- b summer epidemics occur
- c symptoms commonly last longer than one week
- d there is no predictable development of immunity
- e transmission is from infected fowl

(Answers overleaf)

17 b d e
Drugs causing cholestatic jaundice include oestrogens, androgens, chlorpromazine, erythromycin, rifampicin, carbimazole, sulphonamides and nitrofurantoin. Phenacetin produces a haemolytic jaundice and methyldopa may cause jaundice by haemolysis or hepatitis.

18 b d e
Carcinoid tumours are derived from argentaffin cells and tumours which produce the syndrome (flushing, diarrhoea, abdominal pain, wheeze, etc) include appendix, ileum, bronchus and pancreas. The syndrome occurs in $\approx$5% of carcinoids. Hormones produced are 5HT and occasionally ACTH. Diagnosis is by increased urinary 5-hydroxyindoleacetic acid and treatment involves surgery, methysergide and antihistamines. Hepatic artery embolisation is used in some cases.

19 b c d
Gastric cancer is commoner in Japan, in people of blood group A, males>females, chronic gastritis and post-gastrectomy.

20 a d
Norwalk virus infection occurs in all ages and in winter epidemics. Fever, vomiting and abdominal pain are common. Symptoms last about 48 hours and there is no predictable development of immunity. Transmission is from shellfish.

6. Genetics

1. **The following conditions are inherited in an autosomal dominant manner:**
   a. peroneal muscular atrophy
   b. ataxia telangiectasia
   c. arachnodactyly
   d. Friedreich's ataxia
   e. hereditary spherocytosis

2. **The following are characteristic of Klinefelter's syndrome:**
   a. short stature
   b. patients are usually impotent
   c. affected patients are usually born to older mothers
   d. the testes are small but firm
   e. gonadotrophin levels are elevated

3. **Inherited diseases predisposing to malignancy include:**
   a. Fanconi's anaemia
   b. Hurler's syndrome
   c. ataxia telangiectasia
   d. xeroderma pigmentosum
   e. phenylketonuria

4. **Malignant hyperpyrexia:**
   a. is inherited as an autosomal dominant
   b. is associated with a normal creatine phosphokinase level
   c. results in a severe metabolic acidosis
   d. is associated with a 9/22 translocation
   e. may be induced by trichloro-ethylene

5. **The following are features of Turner's syndrome:**
   a. autosomal dominant inheritance
   b. mental retardation is common
   c. elevated gonadotrophin levels
   d. polydactyly
   e. arched palate

(Answers overleaf)

1 a c e
Conditions inherited as autosomal dominants include achondroplasia, facioscapulohumeral dystrophy, peroneal muscular atrophy, Marfan's syndrome and acute intermittent porphyria. Conditions with recessive inheritance include congenital adrenal hyperplasia, albinism, PKU, Hurler's syndrome, Gaucher's syndrome and Friedreich's ataxia.

2 c d e
Klinefelter's syndrome is characterised by XXY karyotype, infertility but not impotence, normal stature, absence of congenital heart defects, hypogonadism, elevated gonadotrophin levels but low/normal testosterone levels.

3 a c d
Fanconi's anaemia is an autosomal recessive condition which leads to a normal blood film initially but progresses to aplastic anaemia later. There are multiple chromosomal abnormalities (?defective DNA repair). If untreated the prognosis is poor. Development of leukaemia is common. In ataxia telangiectasia the increased risk of developing malignancy may be related to chromosome breaks. Xeroderma pigmentosum is autosomal recessive and is characterised by defective DNA repair leading to early skin aging, and a high risk of developing basal cell carcinoma, squamous cell carcinoma and malignant melanoma.

4 a c e
This condition results in widespread muscle rigidity and hyperpyrexia in association with general anaesthesia. It is seen most commonly with the use of halothane and succinyl choline. A family history of sudden death during anaesthesia may be elicited. Dantrolene sodium may be used in prevention.

5 c d e
Turner's syndrome (45,X0) is not associated with maternal age. Features include short stature, primary amenorrhoea, coarctation of the aorta, lack of secondary sexual characteristics, webbed neck, red-green colour blindness, increased gonadotrophin levels and reduced oestrogens.

7. Haematology

1. **Target cells in the peripheral blood are seen in:**
   a. haemoglobin C disease
   b. B12 deficiency
   c. iron deficiency
   d. myelofibrosis
   e. septicaemia

2. **The following statements are correct:**
   a. the half-life of albumin in peripheral blood is 7 days
   b. the life span of a neutrophil is 6 hours
   c. the life span of a red blood cell is 120 days
   d. platelets have a life span of around 10 days
   e. small lymphocytes survive in the peripheral blood for about 100 days

3. **Concerning iron metabolism:**
   a. the total body store of iron is around 40 grams
   b. about half the body's iron is present in haemoglobin
   c. daily iron loss for a male is 0.6 mg
   d. iron is transported in peripheral blood bound to a β-globulin
   e. absorption of iron takes place mainly in the terminal ileum

4. **A dimorphic peripheral blood film is seen in:**
   a. coeliac disease
   b. post-gastrectomy patients
   c. iron deficiency
   d. β thalassaemia
   e. sideroblastic anaemia

5. **Pancytopenia occurs in:**
   a. systemic lupus erythematosus
   b. paroxysmal nocturnal haemoglobinuria
   c. hypersplenism
   d. treatment with nalidixic acid
   e. isoniazid therapy

(Answers overleaf)

1 a c
Target cells may be seen in thalassaemia, iron deficiency, post-splenectomy, haemoglobinopathies and obstructive liver disease. Macrocytes are seen in B12 deficiency and 'tear-drop' cells are found in myelofibrosis.

2 b c d
Albumin is synthesised by the liver and has a molecular weight of 67 000. Levels may fall in liver disease, malnutrition, nephrotic syndrome and severe burns. Its half-life is 21 days.

3 b c d
The total body iron store is around 4–4.5 grams of which about half is present in haemoglobin. Absorption is mainly by the duodenum and jejunum. Iron is transported by transferrin, a β-1 globulin.

4 a b e
Coeliac disease leads to a dimorphic film because of combined iron and B12/folate deficiency. Sideroblastic anaemia may produce either a microcytic or dimorphic picture. Both iron deficiency and thalassaemia result in microcytic anaemias.

5 a b c e
Pancytopenia (anaemia, leucopenia and thrombocytopenia) may be due to aplastic anaemia, hypersplenism, bone marrow infiltration by tumour, megaloblastic anaemia and myelofibrosis.

HAEMATOLOGY

6 The following are true of polycythaemia rubra vera:
   a arterial O_2 saturation may be low
   b B12 levels are decreased
   c erythroid hyperplasia is seen in the bone marrow
   d the neutrophil alkaline phosphatase (NAP) score is decreased
   e bone marrow iron staining is diminished

7 2,3-DPG levels in blood are decreased in:
   a acidosis
   b stored blood
   c anaemia
   d hypopituitarism
   e thyrotoxicosis

8 A patient with acute leukaemia is more likely to have acute myeloid leukaemia as opposed to acute lymphoblastic if:
   a the patient is a child
   b Auer rods are seen
   c cells have >2 nuclei
   d there is a high nucleus:cytoplasm ratio
   e periodic acid-Schiff (PAS) stain is negative

9 Carcino-embryonic antigen (CEA) may be used as a tumour marker for the following conditions:
   a lung cancer
   b ulcerative colitis
   c colonic polyps
   d breast cancer
   e gastrointestinal malignancy

10 The following abnormalities may be seen in the post-splenectomy peripheral blood film:
    a teardrop cell
    b leptocyte
    c Pappenheimer bodies
    d spur cell
    e Howell-Jolly bodies

11 Causes of a monocytosis include:
    a tuberculosis
    b scabies
    c Hodgkin's disease
    d brucellosis
    e myeloma

(Answers overleaf)

6 a c e
Polycythaemia rubra vera is a disease of haemopoietic tissue leading to autonomous proliferation of erythroid, granulocytic or megakaryocytic cell lines. Haemoglobin, red cell count and haematocrit are all elevated. It tends to affect older patients (M = F). B12 levels and B12 binding capacity are elevated as is the NAP score. Complications include hyperviscosity, haemorrhage, thrombosis, hypertension and gout.

7 a b d
An increase in 2,3-DPG results in decreased oxygen affinity of haemoglobin and the oxygen dissociation curve is shifted to the right. Levels are raised in anaemia, heart disease and thyrotoxicosis. Reduced levels are seen in acidosis and stored blood.

8 b c e
AML occurs at all ages but is seen more commonly in adults. Features common to both types of leukaemia (AML and ALL) are anaemia, neutropenia and thrombocytopenia. Lymphoid infiltration is less common than with ALL but gum infiltration is seen more commonly. The peripheral blood film in AML will show myeloblasts which have a low nucleus:cytoplasm ratio, Auer rods and cytoplasmic granules. There are often 3–5 nucleoli.

9 e
CEA is found in fetal pancreas, liver and gut as well as colonic and pancreatic neoplasms. Levels may be used to monitor treatment of certain malignancies but the marker is relatively non-specific.

10 c d e
A post-splenectomy blood film may show spur cells, target cells, increased numbers of platelets, Pappenheimer bodies and Howell-Jolly bodies.

11 a c d
A monocytosis may be due to Hodgkin's disease, monocytic leukaemia, infectious mononucleosis, TB, typhoid, malaria and trypanosomiasis.

HAEMATOLOGY

12 Hyposplenism may be caused by:
a ulcerative colitis
b Fanconi's anaemia
c thalassaemia
d a congenital defect
e tropical sprue

13 Causes of a low ESR include:
a uraemia
b hypofibrinogenaemia
c carcinomatosis
d hypogammaglobulinaemia
e congestive cardiac failure

14 Antithrombin III deficiency may be caused by:
a oestrogens
b Bernard-Soulier disease
c nephrotic syndrome
d thrombasthenia
e liver disease

15 The following statements about methaemoglobinaemia are correct:
a iron is oxidised to the ferrous state
b formation of methaemoglobin is more rapid in children
c cyanosis occurs when more than 10% of the total haemoglobin is methaemoglobin
d formation of methaemoglobin is prevented by glutathione
e improvement is seen with the administration of methylene blue dye

16 In Waldenström's macroglobulinaemia:
a the paraprotein is usually of IgG type
b the condition occurs with roughly equal frequency in men and women
c visual disturbance occurs
d lymph node architecture is destroyed
e an excess of plasmacytoid cells is seen in the bone marrow

17 Chronic granulomatous disease:
a is inherited as an autosomal dominant
b shows no diagnostic changes in the peripheral blood film
c is a disease predominantly of males
d has hepatic abscess as a recognised complication
e is associated with neutrophils which fail to reduce nitroblue tetrazolium dye

(Answers overleaf)

12 a b d e
The blood film in hyposplenism shows target cells and spur cells. Causes include splenectomy, coeliac disease, ulcerative colitis, sickle cell anaemia, Fanconi's anaemia, carcinomatosis and amyloid.

13 b d e
The ESR may be raised in infection, inflammatory conditions, collagen-vascular disease, malignancy, pregnancy, anaemia and hypofibrinogenaemia. Causes of a low ESR include polycythaemia and congestive cardiac failure.

14 a c e
Antithrombin III is synthesised by the liver and inactivates thrombin, factor Xa, VII and plasmin. Heparin owes its actions to antithrombin III. Deficiency occurs with heparin treatment, nephrotic syndrome and liver disease. Bernard-Soulier disease (giant platelets) is unrelated to antithrombin III deficiency and is associated with thrombocytopenia and glycoprotein 1B deficiency.

15 b c d e
Iron is oxidised from the ferrous to ferric form. The formation of methaemoglobin is enhanced in infants since fetal haemoglobin is more susceptible to oxidation. Hypoxic symptoms occur when methaemoglobin constitutes >35% of total haemoglobin; cyanosis occurs when >10% of haemoglobin is methaemoglobin. Methylene blue may be of value in severe methaemoglobinaemia (acquired).

16 c e
This is due to proliferation of lymphocytes, plasmacytoid, lmphocytes and plasma cells. Lymph node architecture is preserved. The condition is commoner in the elderly (M>F). The paraproteinaemia (IgM) leads to hyperviscosity syndrome, heart failure, renal failure and visual disturbance. In 10% cases Bence Jones proteinuria is present. Treatment is with chlorambucil or plasmapharesis.

17 b c d e
This is an X-linked recessive condition in which there is defective intracellular killing of microorganisms. The neutrophils fail to reduce nitroblue tetrazolium dye. It occurs more commonly in boys and is associated with infections, especially of the lungs, liver and bone. Granulocyte transfusions are used in emergencies.

HAEMATOLOGY

18 In von Willebrand's disease:
a the incidence is similar to that of haemophilia
b inheritance is autosomal recessive
c platelet aggregation in response to adrenaline is normal
d there is a reduced level of factor VIII-related antigen
e haemarthrosis is rare

19 Drugs recognised as causing immune haemolytic anaemia include:
a minoxidil
b sulphasalazine
c chlorpropamide
d penicillin
e phenacetin

20 Conditions causing a raised platelet count in the peripheral blood film include:
a myelofibrosis
b patients on vinca alkaloids
c patients receiving corticosteroids
d exercise
e chronic inflammatory bowel disease

21 Haemoglobin A2 ($\alpha 2, \delta 2$) is increased in:
a α thalassaemia
b iron deficiency
c β thalassaemia
d megaloblastic anaemia
e sideroblastic anaemia

22 Drugs which cause haemolysis in patients with glucose-6-phosphate dehydrogenase deficiency include:
a isoniazid
b phenacetin
c penicillin
d chloramphenicol
e erythromycin

23 The presence of ring sideroblasts and excess iron in the bone marrow can be accounted for if the patient has:
a carcinoma
b diabetes mellitus
c polycythaemia rubra vera
d erythropoietic porphyria
e pyridoxine deficiency

(Answers overleaf)

18 a c d e
Von Willebrand's disease is autosomal dominant and is associated with prolongation of the bleeding time, reduced levels of factor VIII-related antigen and factor VIII clotting time. Platelet aggregation with ristocetin is reduced but is normal with ADP and adrenaline. Treatment consists of cryoprecipitate or factor VIII.

19 c d e
Drugs may produce an immune reaction resulting in red cell destruction. Those drugs implicated include chlorpromazine, penicillin, insecticides, sulphonamides, phenacetin and quinidine.

20 b c d e
A raised platelet count may be a consequence of splenectomy, splenic atrophy, malignant disease, vinca alkaloids, steroids, myelofibrosis or polycythaemia rubra vera, amongst others.

21 c d
HbA2 in normal adults is a minor (2% total) haemoglobin. In patients with suspected haemoglobinopathy measurement of the HbA2 concentration may aid in the diagnosis. In β thalassaemia the HbA2 concentration is raised but in α thalassaemia it is *reduced*. In megaloblastic anaemia and unstable haemoglobin disease HbA2 is higher than normal. HbA2 is also decreased in iron deficiency and sideroblastic anaemia.

22 a b c
Haemolysis occurs with a variety of drugs in G6PD deficiency such as antimalarials, sulphonamides, dapsone, nitrofurantoin, nalidixic acid, antihelminthics and quinidine. The degree of haemolysis varies with the drug and concentration used as well as the type of G6PD deficiency the patient is suffering from. Chloramphenicol and erythromycin do not cause haemolysis in these patients.

23 a c d e
Sideroblastic anaemia may be primary or secondary. Secondary causes include vitamin B6 deficiency, anti-tuberculous therapy, coeliac disease, haemolytic anaemia, alcoholism, chloramphenicol, lead poisoning, erythropoietic porphyria, rheumatoid arthritis and carcinoma. This type of anaemia is also associated with myeloproliferative disorders such as polycythaemia rubra vera, acute myeloid leukaemia and myelofibrosis.

24 **The following are associated with a lymphocytosis in the peripheral blood film:**
   a mumps
   b pertussis
   c Kala-azar
   d Hodgkin's disease
   e syphilis

25 **Nucleated red blood cells and granulocyte precursors in the peripheral blood film would be compatible with:**
   a eclampsia
   b miliary tuberculosis
   c thrombotic thrombocytopenic purpura
   d metastatic breast carcinoma
   e Hodgkin's disease

(Answers overleaf)

24 a b e

An absolute lymphocytosis (>3.5 × 10^9/l) occurs in a variety of conditions including glandular fever (atypical lymphocytes), mumps, whooping cough, tuberculosis, syphilis, brucellosis and chronic lymphatic leukaemia. Hodgkin's disease is associated with monocytosis or eosinophilia and Kala-azar is associated with a monocytosis rather than a lymphocytosis.

25 b c d e

A leuco-erythroblastic picture may occur in malignancy, myeloma, myelofibrosis, marble bone disease, Hodgkin's disease, miliary tuberculosis and thrombotic thrombocytopenic purpura. A *leukaemoid reaction* (high leucocyte count in non-leukaemic diseases) may occur in eclampsia, overwhelming infection, burns and neoplasia.

8. Infectious/tropical diseases

1 **The following incubation periods are correct:**
   a cholera   2–3 hours
   b mumps   1–7 days
   c rubella   14–21 days
   d hepatitis A   2–6 weeks
   e anthrax   7–14 days

2 **The following are live vaccines:**
   a yellow fever
   b hepatitis B
   c polio
   d diphtheria
   e pertussis

3 **Cholera toxin:**
   a has 'A', 'B' and 'C' subunits
   b promotes an increase in intracellular cAMP
   c 'A' subunits are responsible for mucosal attachment
   d inhibits sodium and chloride reabsorption in villus cells
   e induces no inflammatory changes in the bowel

4 **In typhoid fever:**
   a the white blood count is decreased with a relative lymphopenia
   b stool culture is positive in the first week
   c blood culture is positive in the first week
   d the organism can be grown from bone marrow after blood cultures have become negative
   e antibiotic treatment is not always necessary

(Answers overleaf)

1 a c d
Mumps has an incubation of 12–21 days and anthrax has a short incubation period of 2–5 days. Diseases with long incubation periods include hepatitis B (6 weeks–6 months), leprosy (months–years) and rabies (2–8 weeks).

2 a c
Live vaccines are polio, measles, rubella, smallpox and yellow fever. These should not be given in pregnancy, during an acute febrile illness, with other live vaccines and to patients on steroids.

3 b d e
Cholera is caused by toxogenic strains of *Vibrio cholerae* which produces toxin (A and B subunits). The toxin activates adenyl cyclase producing a severe secretory diarrhoea. Hypovolaemia and hypokalaemia may result. Treatment is with fluid/electrolyte replacement. Oral tetracycline may be used in the acute illness and in asymptomatic carriers.

4 c d
In typhoid fever the white blood count is usually low with neutropenia. The organism may be cultured from blood in the first 7 to 10 days and from stool in the third to fourth week. Stool/urine cultures are less helpful than blood culture in the diagnosis and, although stool cultures are mandatory, they are not often positive when blood culture is negative in early typhoid. Patients suspected of suffering from typhoid should be barrier-nursed and intravenous fluids/electrolytes should be given. Antibiotic therapy should be started with amoxycillin, ampicillin or cotrimoxazole.

INFECTIOUS/TROPICAL DISEASES

5 **The following statements regarding antibacterial drugs are true:**
   a aminoglycosides inhibit production of mRNA
   b tetracyclines interfere with cell wall synthesis
   c sulphonamides interfere with bacterial folate synthesis
   d quinolones act by preventing tRNA synthesis
   e tobramycin is less active against *Pseudomonas* than gentamicin

6 **The following statements about the AIDS virus are correct:**
   a the virus is a rubivirus
   b the genome is composed of RNA
   c reverse transcriptase is present in the virus core
   d affected individuals are only infectious when their immune system is impaired
   e deterioration, clinically, correlates with loss of demonstrable antibody to the core protein of the virus

7 **DNA viruses include:**
   a orthomyxoviruses
   b rhinovirus
   c infectious mononucleosis
   d cytomegalovirus
   e herpes virus

8 **Diseases leading to neutropenia include:**
   a brucellosis
   b systemic lupus erythematosus
   c scarlet fever
   d anthrax
   e typhoid

9 **Glandular fever:**
   a causes a maculopapular rash most prominent on flexor surfaces
   b may lead to an abnormal ECG
   c has splenic rupture as a known complication
   d infection may lead to cranial nerve lesions
   e infection is due to an RNA virus

10 **Measles:**
   a is due to a DNA virus
   b may lead to an abnormal EEG in later life
   c has its most infective period around the rash stage
   d infection is associated with myoclonic jerks
   e may be associated with gastroenteritis as part of the initial illness

(Answers overleaf)

5 a c
Tetracyclines interfere with the 30s subunit of bacterial ribosomes preventing mRNA translation. Tobramycin is more active than gentamicin against *Pseudomonas*.

6 b c e
The AIDS virus is a so-called lentivirus and has RNA as its genetic material. Reverse transcriptase is an enzyme which makes DNA copies from an RNA template. Affected individuals are most infectious when they are first infected and later when their immune systems fail. During these two periods it is easiest to demonstrate the presence of the virus.

7 c d e
Pox, herpes, adenovirus, Epstein Barr virus (infectious mononucleosis) and cytomegalovirus are DNA viruses. RNA viruses include enteroviruses (polio, coxsackie and echo), paramyxoviruses, orthomyxoviruses, rhabdovirus, rubella, hepatitis A and rhinovirus.

8 a b e
Neutropenia may be a feature of infection with yellow fever, brucella, typhoid, Lassa fever, influenza, Marburg virus and conditions such as SLE and myelofibrosis.

9 b c d
This is caused by infection by Epstein-Barr virus. The rash is maculopapular and occurs predominantly on extensor surfaces. Myocarditis is a feature and leads to ECG abnormalities. Other complications include glomerulonephritis, meningo-encephalitis, cranial/peripheral nerve lesions, autoimmune haemolytic anaemia, thrombocytopenia and Guillain-Barré syndrome.

10 b d e
Measles is a paramyxovirus (RNA). The EEG may be abnormal if subacute sclerosing panencephalitis develops some years later. The most infective period is the catarrhal stage. Complications include convulsions, otitis media, pneumonia, gastroenteritis and encephalitis.

INFECTIOUS/TROPICAL DISEASES

11 Legionnaire's disease is associated with:
  a lymphocytosis
  b peak incidence in winter
  c cigarette smoking
  d higher attack rate than Pontiac fever
  e infection with a gram positive coccobacillus

12 Whooping cough:
  a is a notifiable disease
  b is a recognised cause of subdural haematoma
  c is associated with lymphopenia
  d is caused by a gram positive bacterium
  e vaccination is with a killed virus

13 Anthrax:
  a has an incubation period of 7–21 days
  b is associated with a painful 'malignant pustule'
  c may lead to cerebral thrombosis
  d is due to a gram positive spore-bearing bacterium
  e is associated with a relative neutropenia

14 Characteristic features of brucellosis include:
  a arthritis affecting small joints
  b neutropenia
  c raised white blood cell count
  d depression
  e sterile pyuria

15 Salmonella food poisoning:
  a occurs 2–6 hours after ingestion of contaminated food
  b is particularly severe in patients with pernicious anaemia
  c is due to production of enterotoxin
  d is not associated with a carrier state
  e may be associated with bloody diarrhoea

16 Trichinosis is associated with:
  a basophilia on the peripheral blood film
  b periorbital oedema
  c urticaria
  d polyneuritis
  e resolution with thiabendazole

(Answers overleaf)

11 c
Legionnaire's disease is caused by a gram negative coccobacillus. The white blood count is raised with a neutrophilia. Peak incidence is in summer and the disease has a lower attack rate than Pontiac fever (Legionnaire's without the pneumonia). Complications include headache, myalgia, abdominal pain, meningitis, encephalitis, neuropathy, hepatitis and confusion.

12 a b e
Whooping cough is caused by the gram negative bacterium *Bordetella pertussis*. It affects mainly children under 5 years of age and most deaths are seen in infants less than 6 months old. There is no placental immunity. Lymphocytosis occurs and diagnosis is made by pernasal swabs. Complications include pneumonia, bronchiectasis, fits, subconjunctival haemorrhage, rectal prolapse and secondary bacterial infection.

13 c d
Anthrax is caused by a gram positive spore-bearing bacterium, *Bacillus anthracis*. The infection has a short incubation period of 1–3 days and is due to inhalation of spores. Malignant pustules are seen but these are characteristically painless. The white blood cells show neutrophilia.

14 a b d e
Brucellosis is due to infection by a gram negative rod. The white blood count is not raised and there is relative neutropenia. Symptoms include spondylitis, sweating, rigors, depression and arthritis. Treatment is with tetracycline for 3 weeks.

15 b e
Salmonella food poisoning is due to a gram negative bacterium and produces symptoms after 12–48 hours. Infection is usually from meat or fowl and may be particularly severe in patients with pernicious anaemia. Symptoms are due to gut invasion and not enterotoxin. Use of antibiotics may prolong the carrier state and should be avoided if possible.

16 b c d e
This is caused by the nematode *Trichinella spiralis*. Cysts are ingested in undercooked pork. The incubation period is 2 days followed by nausea, abdominal pain and diarrhoea. Allergic reactions are common and patients develop myalgia, fever, eosinophilia, urticaria and facial oedema. Treatment is with thiabendazole. Steroids may be used to control symptoms due to allergic reactions.

INFECTIOUS/TROPICAL DISEASES

17 In cryptococcal infection:
a respiratory symptoms are less common than those of the central nervous system
b gummatous lesions are seen in bone
c meningitis is common
d the disease is spread mainly from infected pork
e the organism is a gram negative bacterium

18 The following statements regarding Leptospirosis are true:
a it is a zoonosis
b infection leads to renal and liver failure
c CSF protein may be normal
d blood culture becomes positive from the second week of the illness
e meningitis is rare

19 In melioidosis:
a a gram positive bacterium is responsible
b diagnosis is by agglutination with a specific antiserum
c perinephric abscess is a common complication
d the condition occurs in cattle and pigs
e granulomas which resemble those of tuberculosis occur

20 Kala-azar is associated with:
a lymphocytosis
b positive spleen smear
c hypergammaglobulinaemia
d double daily temperature spike
e hyperpigmented skin lesions

21 Tuberculoid as opposed to lepromatous leprosy:
a is non-infective
b is associated with a negative Lepromin test
c shows no cell-mediated immune response
d shows no organisms in skin patches
e shows a marked tuberculoid response

(Answers overleaf)

17 a b c
Cryptococcal infection is commoner in patients with disordered cell-mediated immunity. The organism *Cryptococcus neoformans* is a yeast and produces a meningitis-like illness. Neurological symptoms are commonest and granulomatous reactions are found in the lungs, bone, brain and meninges. Diagnosis is from CSF culture, identification of spores and serology. Amphoteracin ±flucytosine are used in treatment.

18 a c
Leptospira icterohaemorrhagiae is found in rat urine and humans are infected from contaminated water. Weil's disease is the most serious form. The incubation period is 2–4 weeks after which time patients are prostrated with high fever, headache, myalgia and jaundice. Diagnosis is by serology of paired sera. Renal failure rather than liver failure may result and treatment is with benzylpenicillin.

19 b d e
This tropical disease is due to infection with *Pseudomonas pseudomallei*, a gram negative bacterium. The organism produces endo- and exotoxins. Melioidosis has been described in a variety of animals including cattle, pigs, rodents and kangaroos. Clinical features are wide ranging and include pneumonitis, granulomas, septic arthritis, liver abscess, pericarditis and septicaemia. Perinephric abscess does occur but it is not common. Treatment may be with a variety of antibiotics including cotrimoxazole, tetracyclines and chloramphenicol.

20 b c d
Kala-azar (Leishmaniasis) is transmitted by the sandfly *Phlebotomus*. The incubation period is 1–2 months. Raised gamma globulin, massive splenomegaly and double-daily temperature spike are characteristic. Leucopenia, anaemia, thrombocytopenia and hypoalbuminaemia may be found. Skin may show decreased pigmentation.

21 a d e
Tuberculoid leprosy produces hypopigmented areas of skin, marked tuberculoid response, thickened peripheral nerves and positive Lepromin test, and organisms are absent from skin patches. Lepromatous leprosy shows no cell-mediated response (no tuberculoid response), bacilli numerous in skin lesions, leonine facies, Charcot joints and glove-and-stocking sensory loss.

INFECTIOUS/TROPICAL DISEASES

22 Conditions leading to persistently false-positive syphilis serology include:
  a tuberculosis
  b Reiter's disease
  c malaria
  d bejel
  e rheumatoid arthritis

23 Features of *Toxocara* infection include:
  a splenomegaly
  b epilepsy as a complication
  c asthma
  d low IgE levels
  e subclinical cases are unusual

24 *Chlamydia* are responsible for:
  a ornithosis
  b bagassosis
  c lymphogranuloma venereum
  d rectal stricture
  e neonatal eye infection

25 Isoniazid toxicity includes:
  a antagonism of the oral contraceptive pill
  b systemic lupus erythematosus
  c hepatitis
  d potentiation of warfarin
  e increased toxicity in pregnancy

(Answers overleaf)

22 b d e
Conditions which may lead to persistently false-positive serology (i.e. longer than 6 months) include SLE, yaws, leprosy, pinta, bejel, Reiter's syndrome, rheumatoid arthritis, other autoimmune conditions and narcotic addiction. Serology may be transiently positive in malaria, tuberculosis, glandular fever and mycoplasma pneumonias.

23 a b c
Toxocara canis (dog nematode) infection is common in children and leads to asthma, eosinophilia, splenomegaly and sometimes blindness due to the presence of dead larvae in the eye. There is raised IgE/IgM and generalised lymphadenopathy. Epilepsy is a recognised complication and treatment is with thiabendazole.

24 a c d e
These organisms cause a variety of conditions such as psittacosis, ornithosis, non-specific urethritis, cat-scratch fever, lymphogranuloma venereum and trachoma. Bagassosis is one type of extrinsic allergic alveolitis.

25 b c d e
Side effects of isoniazid include hepatitis, SLE, pyridoxine deficiency, pellagra-like rash, insomnia, muscle twitching, neuropathy and optic neuritis. It potentiates phenytoin and warfarin. Rifampicin antagonises warfarin and the oral contraceptive pill.

9. Metabolic disease

1 **The following statements about Paget's disease of bone are true:**
   a   The condition is rare in Orientals
   b   a raised urinary hydroxyproline level is found
   c   the condition may present with tunnel vision
   d   it is commoner in males than females
   e   less than 5% of sufferers have symptoms

2 **Elevated serum acid phosphatase is found in:**
   a   Von Gierke's disease (type I glycogen storage disease)
   b   osteogenic sarcoma
   c   scurvy
   d   Gaucher's disease (β-glucosidase deficiency)
   e   hyperparathyroidism

3 **The following statements about renal tubular acidosis (RTA) are true:**
   a   the urine pH is always above 5.4 in distal RTA
   b   the condition may be acquired as part of the Fanconi syndrome
   c   an acid urine can be produced in distal but not proximal RTA
   d   vitamin D resistant rickets may result from the chronic acidosis
   e   hypervitaminosis D predisposes to proximal RTA

4 **Homocystinuria:**
   a   is inherited in an autosomal dominant manner
   b   presents with renal calculi
   c   results in lens dislocation
   d   predisposes to thrombo-embolism
   e   results in mental retardation

(Answers overleaf)

1 a b c e
The incidence of Paget's disease of bone increases with age. The aetiology is unknown and it is associated with a raised serum alkaline phosphatase but normal calcium and phosphate unless immobilised. If alkaline phosphatase levels rise unexpectedly osteosarcoma should be suspected. Other complications are high output heart failure, pathological fracture and closure of skull foramina (deafness, etc).

2 b d e
Acid phosphatase is found in several tissues including red blood cells, prostate and bone. In prostatic carcinoma acid phosphatase rises because of the increased number of cells making it. Other causes include: urinary retention, catheterisation and Gaucher's disease.

3 a b d e
RTA may be inherited or acquired (vitamin D deficiency, nephrotic syndrome, myeloma, amphoteracin B and renal transplant rejection). The two main groups are: *distal* (classical) and *proximal* depending on the site. In distal RTA the hydrogen transport mechanism is defective and the urine is not acidified. In proximal RTA the tubular reabsorption of HCO_3 is impaired. Other features include hyperchloraemia, hypokalaemia and renal calculi.

4 c d e
This condition resembles Marfan's syndrome. There is osteoporosis, downwards lens dislocation (cf Marfan's), mental retardation and increased incidence of atherothrombotic disease. Treatment is with pyridoxine, cystine and methionine restriction.

METABOLIC DISEASES

5 **The following statements regarding abetalipoproteinaemia are correct:**
   a inheritance is autosomal recessive
   b steatorrhoea may be a presenting feature
   c ataxia may be present
   d serum lipids are elevated
   e retinitis pigmentosa is recognised

6 **In acute intermittent porphyria:**
   a urinary 5-amino laevulinate is elevated
   b pregnancy may be dangerous
   c glucose infusion makes an attack worse
   d the enzyme defect is uroporphyrinogen-1-synthetase
   e hyponatraemia occurs

7 **Features characteristic of Wilson's disease include:**
   a osteoporosis
   b low urinary copper
   c low serum copper
   d osteoarthritis
   e phosphaturia

8 **Causes of osteomalacia include:**
   a coeliac disease
   b hypothyroidism
   c renal tubular acidosis
   d Fanconi syndrome
   e chronic liver disease

9 **In haemochromatosis:**
   a iron is deposited in Kupffer cells of the liver
   b hepatoma is a recognised cause of death
   c arthropathy affecting predominantly small joints is a feature
   d skin pigmentation is due solely to iron deposition
   e clinical diabetes is present in a minority of cases

10 **The following proteins rise in concentration in response to tissue damage:**
   a fibrinogen
   b pre-albumin
   c transferrin
   d α-2 globulins
   e C-reactive protein

(Answers overleaf)

5 a b c e
This condition results in impaired chylomicron and VLDL synthesis. Transport of lipid from the gut to liver is impaired. Other findings include retinitis pigmentosa, acanthocytosis and ataxia.

6 a b d e
The porphyrias are inherited disorders of porphyrin metabolism. There are six main types and each one has a specific enzyme defect. In AIP the defect is in uroporphyrinogen-1-synthetase and inheritance is autosomal dominant. Skin lesions never occur but acute attacks may be precipitated by barbiturates, fasting, alcohol and intercurrent infection. Glucose infusion may be used to treat an attack. AIP is also a cause of inappropriate ADH secretion.

7 a c d e
Wilson's disease (hepatolenticular degeneration) is inherited as an autosomal recessive. The basic defect is decreased serum caeruloplasmin which leads to low plasma copper levels and copper deposition in the kidneys, basal ganglia, liver and cornea. Urinary copper is elevated. Treatment is with penicillamine.

8 a c d e
Osteomalacia (adult rickets) may be due to vitamin D deficiency or resistance. Deficiency occurs in conditions with insufficient sunlight, poor diet or malabsorption. Vitamin D resistance is found in chronic renal failure, anticonvulsant therapy and liver disease. Biochemical features are hypocalcaemia, low or normal serum phosphate and raised alkaline phosphatase.

9 b
Haemochromatosis (bronze diabetes) is inherited as an autosomal recessive. Oral iron absorption is elevated. Cirrhosis/varices may occur. Hypogonadism and heart failure are features and diabetes results due to iron deposition in the pancreas. The skin is pigmented because of increased pigmentary iron and melanin.

10 a d e
In tissue trauma (including infection and malignancy) acute phase reactants increase in serum. These include C-reactive protein, α-1 and α-2 globulins and fibrinogen. Conversely, there are some proteins which decrease in concentration including pre-albumin, albumin and transferrin. The rise in acute phase reactants is relatively non-specific.

METABOLIC DISEASES

11 Causes of hypophosphataemia include:
  a insulin treatment in diabetic ketoacidosis
  b osteoporosis
  c Paget's disease of bone
  d severe burns
  e tertiary hyperparathyroidism

12 The following are recognised in hypothermia:
  a metabolic alkalosis
  b lack of shivering
  c pancreatitis
  d hyperkalaemia
  e delta wave on ECG

13 5'-nucleotidase:
  a is found in thyroid
  b levels are reduced in liver disease
  c levels are normal in bone disease
  d levels are unaffected by enzyme inducers
  e deficiency occurs in some cases of adult acquired hypogammaglobulinaemia

14 Osteoporosis is associated with:
  a cigarette smoking
  b hypothyroidism
  c caffeine
  d obesity
  e alcoholism

15 The following findings would support a diagnosis of anorexia nervosa:
  a low cholesterol levels
  b reduced follicle stimulating hormone (FSH) levels
  c low prolactin levels
  d increased cortisol
  e atrophy of breast tissue in females

16 The following conditions predispose to metabolic acidosis with an anion gap between 8 and 12:
  a diabetic ketoacidosis
  b renal tubular acidosis
  c diarrhoea
  d acetazolamide therapy
  e methanol-induced acidosis

(Answers overleaf)

11 a d e

Hypophosphataemia may lead to rickets (Familial Hypophosphataemic Rickets) and this is an X-linked condition due to impaired tubular reabsorption of phosphate. Severe burns and hyperparathyroidism both lead to lowered serum phosphate. Hypophosphataemia is usually due to excess parathormone. With insulin treatment phosphate enters the cells (i.e. acts like potassium). Parenteral feeding with inadequate replacement may also lead to a similar picture.

12 b c d

Other features include: 'J' waves on ECG, arrhythmias, metabolic acidosis, hyperkalaemia and pancreatitis.

13 a c d e

Serum 5'-nucleotidase is increased in biliary tract obstruction but is not one of the inducible liver enzymes. Its function is to catalyse the hydrolysis of nucleotides which have phosphate in the pentose sugar in the 5' position.

14 a c e

In osteoporosis bone mass is reduced but the remaining bone is of normal composition. Biochemically, unlike osteomalacia, the serum phosphate, calcium and alkaline phosphatase are normal. Causes include post-menopause, Cushing's disease, hypogonadism and alcoholism.

15 b d

In anorexia the following may be found:
Normal: thyroid function, amino acids, vitamins and prolactin levels
Low: serum K^+, FSH and LH
High: serum cortisol, growth hormone and cholesterol. There is increased lanugo hair and breast tissue atrophy is *not* a feature.

16 b c d

One must first list the causes of metabolic acidosis and discount those with a high anion gap (e.g. diabetic ketoacidosis, lactic acidosis). The anion gap may be calculated by:

$$([Na^+] + [K^+]) - ([Cl^-] + [HCO_3^-])$$

Those conditions which produce a normal gap acidosis include: renal tubular acidosis, high intestinal fistulae, acetazolamide therapy and transplantation of the ureter into the colon (a procedure which is not performed now).

METABOLIC DISEASES

17 The following statements about hyperlipidaemias are true:
  a familial hypercholesterolaemia is inherited as an autosomal dominant
  b type III hyperlipidaemia is due to Apo E-III deficiency plus familial combined hyperlipidaemia
  c type IV hyperlipidaemia is associated with a clear serum
  d LDL is increased in type IV hyperlipidaemia
  e cholesterol levels are raised in type IIa hyperlipidaemia

18 Fanconi's syndrome is associated with:
  a osteomalacia
  b a defect in the proximal convoluted tubule of the kidney
  c excretion of immunoglobulin light chains
  d adult cystinosis
  e hyperphosphaturia

19 Hypercalcaemia is recognised in:
  a tuberculosis
  b osteoblastic metastases
  c hypoalbuminaemia
  d thyrotoxicosis
  e acromegaly

20 Drugs which are unsafe in acute porphyria include:
  a flufenamic acid
  b gold
  c chlorpromazine
  d probenecid
  e lignocaine

(Answers overleaf)

17 a b e
The WHO classification divides hyperlipidaemias into six main groups. Increasing age is associated with higher levels of serum cholesterol and triglycerides. Hyperlipidaemias may be secondary to other diseases or conditions such as raised cholesterol in diabetes mellitus, pregnancy, porphyria and the nephrotic syndrome. Triglycerides may be raised in obesity, alcoholism and diabetes mellitus. There is no easy way of remembering the details of the hyperlipidaemias and they should be committed to memory for the exam.

18 a b c e
This syndrome is due to a generalised renal tubular transport mechanism defect. Consequences include: osteomalacia (rickets), renal glycosuria, phosphaturia and amino-aciduria.

19 a d e
Hypercalcaemia may be due to bone resorption, primary hyperparathyroidism, thyrotoxicosis, acromegaly, tuberculosis, sarcoidosis, diuretics (thiazides especially). Paget's disease, Milk–Alkali syndrome and vitamin D intoxication. Osteoblastic metastases and hypoalbuminaemia are causes of hypocalcaemia.

20 a b d e
Safe drugs include: pethidine, chlorpromazine, penicillin, aspirin and diazepam. *Unsafe drugs* include: barbiturates, carbamazepine, sulphonamides and griseofulvin.

10. Neurology

1. **The following statements regarding cerebrospinal fluid (CSF) are correct:**
   a. CSF pressure is greater than venous pressure
   b. the rate of formation is 0.5 ml/minute
   c. the pressure is constant
   d. there is a potential difference between CSF and blood of +5 mV
   e. choroid plexus cells secrete 5-hydroxytryptamine into the bloodstream

2. **Autonomic neuropathy may result as a consequence of:**
   a. corticostriatal degeneration
   b. thallium toxicity
   c. Chagas' disease
   d. familial dysautonomia
   e. botulism

3. **Causes of a spastic paraparesis include:**
   a. anterior spinal artery thrombosis
   b. Refsum's disease
   c. syphilis
   d. syringomyelia
   e. B12 deficiency

4. **Muscle fasciculation occurs in:**
   a. hypothyroidism
   b. syphilitic amyotrophy
   c. cervical spondylosis
   d. Charcot-Marie-Tooth disease
   e. multiple sclerosis

(Answers overleaf)

1 b c d e
CSF is produced by cells of the choroid plexus at a rate of ≈0.5 ml/minute. The total volume of CSF is ≈120 ml and is at a pH of 7.33 with a potential difference between CSF and blood of +5 mV. Choroid plexus cells secrete 5-hydroxytryptamine and adrenaline into the bloodstream.

2 a b c d e
In Shy Drager syndrome (corticostriatal degeneration) there is postural hypotension, anhidrosis, impotence, sphincter disturbance and pupillary abnormalities. Familial dysautonomia (Riley Day syndrome) is autosomal recessive and leads to postural hypotension and hyperthermia from birth.

3 a c d e
Spastic paraparesis may be due to multiple sclerosis, trauma, cord compression, motor neurone disease, subacute combined degeneration of the cord, taboparesis, syringomyelia, anterior spinal artery thrombosis and Friedreich's ataxia. In the legs there are signs of an upper motor neurone lesion with increased tone, weakness, ankle clonus and extensor plantars.

4 b c d
Muscle fasciculation occurs classically in a lower motor neurone lesion but may also be seen in cervical spondylosis, thyrotoxicosis, syphilis, Charcot-Marie-Tooth disease and syringomyelia.

NEUROLOGY

5 The following are true of an ulnar nerve lesion:
  a weakness of abduction and adduction of the fingers occurs
  b cervical rib is a recognised cause
  c carcinoma may be the underlying cause
  d there is flexion at the metacarpophalangeal joints and extension at the interphalangeal joints of the fourth and fifth fingers
  e pronation of the forearm is affected

6 Diseases which may have Parkinsonian features include:
  a hyperparathyroidism
  b Wilson's disease
  c Alzheimer's disease
  d normal pressure hydrocephalus
  e olivopontinocerebellar degeneration

7 Features of myotonic dystrophy include:
  a notched QRS on ECG
  b lack of secondary sexual characteristics
  c short QT interval on ECG
  d diabetes mellitus
  e autosomal recessive inheritance

8 In facioscapulohumeral dystrophy:
  a movements of smiling/closing eye are impaired
  b winging of the scapulae occurs
  c inheritance is X-linked recessive
  d the upper half of the face is affected initially
  e cardiomyopathy is not a feature

9 In a patient with neurological symptoms/signs, Friedreich's ataxia is more likely than multiple sclerosis if the following are found:
  a extensor plantars
  b Rombergism
  c preservation of knee and ankle jerks
  d a positive family history
  e normal pain and deep pressure sensation

10 The following statements about dysphasia are true:
  a expressive dysphasia is associated with lesions of the dominant inferior frontal gyrus
  b the prognosis for recovery in global dyphasia is poor
  c lesions leading to nominal dysphasia include those of the dominant inferior temporal gyrus
  d a patient who speaks in neologisms may have normal comprehension
  e the arcuate fasciculus links areas responsible for receptive and expressive speech

(Answers overleaf)

5 a b c
In an ulnar nerve lesion (C7-8, T1) there is weakness and wasting of the small muscles of the hand with thenar sparing. Sensation will be diminished in the ulnar distribution (fifth and medial half of the fourth finger as well as the medial half of the palm). There will be hyperextension at the metacarpophalangeal joints and flexion of the interphalangeal joints producing the so-called 'claw hand'. The affected muscles are flexor carpi ulnaris, medial half of flexor digitorum profundus, the interossei, third and fourth lumbricals, all the hypothenar muscles and adductor pollicis.

6 b c d e
Conditions which show features of Parkinsonism include normal pressure hydrocephalus (incontinence, ataxia and dementia), Alzheimer's disease, Shy Drager syndrome, Wilson's disease, Jakob Creuzfeldt syndrome and hypoparathyroidism (calcification of the basal ganglia).

7 a d
This is inherited as an autosomal dominant and involves the facial muscles, temporalis and masseters. Cataract, balding, ptosis and testicular atrophy are associated. There is diminished IgG and high circulating gonadotrophin levels.

8 a b e
The face is unlined and lacks expression with associated facial and limb girdle wasting. The scapulae may be winged. Inheritance is autosomal dominant and the disease may be relatively benign.

9 b d
The plantars are extensor in both conditions and Rombergism may be present in Friedreich's ataxia but not multiple sclerosis. In Friedreich's the knee and ankle jerks are absent and pain and deep pressure sensation are normal in both.

10 a b d e
Dysphasia is associated with a lesion of the dominant hemisphere which, for most people, is the left; in 25% of left-handed people the dominant hemisphere is the right. Global dysphasia implies damage to a large portion of the dominant hemisphere and hence the prognosis is poor. Nominal dysphasia is believed to be due to a lesion of the posterior part of the superior temporal gyrus.

11 In myasthenia gravis:
  a electromyographic response to ulnar nerve stimulation shows a characteristic rise in amplitude
  b tendon reflexes are absent
  c there is an association with hypothyroidism
  d the presence of a thymoma indicates a better prognosis
  e deterioration has been shown to occur in pregnancy

12 The following are true of syringomyelia:
  a reflexes in the legs are exaggerated
  b pseudobulbar palsy is a feature
  c position sense is retained
  d hydrocephalus occurs in about 25% of cases
  e sphincter disturbance is common

13 In subacute combined degeneration of the cord:
  a the patient may not be anaemic
  b ankle jerks are preserved
  c demyelination is mild
  d optic atrophy occurs
  e dementia is rare

14 The following are recognised features of the lateral medullary syndrome:
  a loss of taste
  b contralateral spinothalamic signs
  c the descending sympathetic tract is involved on the same side as the lesion
  d contralateral IX and X nerve lesions are present
  e the nucleus of the V nerve is affected on the opposite side to the lesion

15 Prolongation of the ankle jerk is seen in:
  a neurosyphilis
  b amyotrophic lateral sclerosis
  c hepatic coma
  d sarcoidosis
  e hypokalaemia

(Answers overleaf)

11 c e
This is a disease affecting the motor endplate with antibodies to acetylcholine receptors. Associated auto-antibodies are rheumatoid factor, antinuclear factor, antimitochondrial antibodies and antismooth muscle antibodies. It is associated with pernicious anaemia, Sjögren's syndrome, hypo- and hyperthyroidism. Diagnosis is with the Tensilon test (edrophonium). Tendon reflexes may be normal or increased. The EMG shows a decrease in amplitude in myasthenia and an increase in the Eaton-Lambert syndrome.

12 a c d
The signs found in syringomyelia are small muscle wasting in the hand, absent reflexes in the upper limbs, dissociated sensory loss and burns and scars on the hand (loss of pain and temperature). A Horner's syndrome may be present and reflexes in the legs are increased with extensor plantars. Bulbar rather than pseudobulbar palsy may be present. Sphincter disturbance is uncommon in syringomyelia.

13 a d e
This is due to B12 deficiency resulting in posterior and lateral column degeneration. Megaloblastic anaemia is usually found but the peripheral blood film may be normal. There is numbness and distal limb weakness and the lower limbs eventually become spastic with extensor plantars. There is loss of vibration and proprioception and well as a 'glove-and-stocking' sensory loss. Demyelination is marked and may precede axonal loss.

14 a b c
The lateral medullary syndrome occurs as a result of posterior inferior cerebellar artery occlusion leading to ipsilateral Horner's syndrome, cerebellar signs, diminished pain and temperature sensation of the face and palatal paralysis. There is contralateral loss of pain and temperature sensation in the trunk and limbs and taste loss is recognised. Patients usually present with diplopia, vertigo, nystagmus, nausea and vomiting.

15 a d e
A prolonged ankle jerk may be seen (classically) in hypothyroidism. Other causes are obesity, sarcoidosis, neurosyphilis, myasthenia, diabetes mellitus and Parkinson's disease. Tendon reflexes may be increased in upper motor neurone lesions as well as multiple sclerosis, amyotrophic lateral sclerosis, thyrotoxicosis and hepatic coma.

NEUROLOGY

16 Signs of a lesion in the parietal lobe include:
  a constructional apraxia
  b urinary incontinence
  c auditory hallucinations
  d prosopagnosia
  e joint position loss

17 Benign intracranial hypertension is associated with:
  a papilloedema
  b anaemia
  c hypercapnia
  d ataxia
  e headache

18 Conditions leading to a predominantly motor peripheral neuropathy include:
  a relapsing idiopathic polyneuropathy
  b carcinomatosis
  c Charcot-Marie-Tooth disease
  d vincristine toxicity
  e porphyria

19 In hypokalaemic periodic paralysis:
  a attacks of flaccid weakness of voluntary muscle occur, including those of speech
  b the symptoms may improve with acetazolamide
  c a non-familial variety occurs in some patients with hyperthyroidism
  d inheritance is autosomal dominant
  e attacks become worse with advancing age

20 Conditions leading to a markedly elevated CSF protein level include:
  a amyloidosis
  b hypothyroidism
  c alcoholism
  d spinal block
  e pyogenic meningitis

(Answers overleaf)

16 a d e
Impaired parietal lobe function leads to disturbed postural sensation, passive movement, two-point discrimination, astereognosis and perceptual rivalry. Gerstmann's syndrome is due to a lesion of the dominant parietal lobe which leads to left/right disorientation, finger agnosia, acalculia and agraphia.

17 a b c e
Benign intracranial hypertension results in headache, papilloedema and diminished acuity usually in obese females. Associations include the oral contraceptive pill, SLE, Behçet's syndrome and hypoparathyroidism. Repeated lumbar puncture may be necessary.

18 a c e
A motor neuropathy is seen in lead poisoning, porphyria, Guillain-Barré syndrome, Charcot-Marie-Tooth disease and relapsing idiopathic polyneuropathy. Sensory neuropathies are associated with diabetes mellitus, carcinoma and vincristine toxicity.

19 b c d
This condition is autosomal dominant and affects patients in their second decade. Exacerbating factors include cold weather and ingestion of food. The bulbar and respiratory muscles are unaffected. Treatment is with potassium supplements in the acute phase and acetazolamide and a high potassium diet for prophylaxis.

20 a c d e
CSF protein may be raised in Guillain-Barré syndrome, spinal block (Froin's syndrome), meningioma, acoustic neuroma, tuberculosis, carcinoma and amyloidosis.

11. Ophthalmology

1. **The following are causes of a large pupil:**
   a. Holmes-Adie syndrome
   b. congenital syphilis
   c. acute iritis
   d. myotonic dystrophy
   e. botulism

2. **The following fundal findings suggest proliferative rather than background diabetic retinopathy:**
   a. micro-aneurysms
   b. soft exudates
   c. flame-shaped haemorrhages
   d. hard exudates
   e. preretinal haemorrhages

3. **Retinal vein thrombosis is associated with:**
   a. papilloedema
   b. diabetes mellitus
   c. hypertension
   d. glaucoma
   e. soft exudates

4. **Retinitis pigmentosa is associated with:**
   a. constriction of the visual fields
   b. Usher's syndrome
   c. Friedreich's ataxia
   d. choroideremia
   e. increased incidence of cataract

5. **In papilloedema as opposed to papillitis there is:**
   a. central scotoma
   b. constricted visual field
   c. normal acuity
   d. tenderness on moving the eye
   e. loss of venous pulsation

(Answers overleaf)

1 a b e
In the Holmes-Adie syndrome the pupils are large and slow-reacting. A large pupil may also be seen with emotion or pain, third nerve lesions and infections such as botulism and diphtheria.

2 b c e
Features of background retinopathy include: micro-aneurysms, dot and blot haemorrhages and hard exudates. Proliferative retinopathy is distinguished by new vessel formation, macular oedema, preretinal haemorrhages, subhyaloid haemorrhage and soft exudates.

3 a b c d e
Retinal vein thrombosis is the most common (after diabetic eye disease) vascular disease of the retina associated with loss of vision. It is associated with hyperviscosity (Waldenström's macroglobulinaemia and myeloma), diabetes mellitus, glaucoma and hypertension. Fundoscopic findings include flame-shaped haemorrhages, cotton wool spots and retinal oedema. If neovascularisation is present then photocoagulation is indicated.

4 a b c e
The fundal appearance resembles bone spicules. It may occur in isolation and transmission is autosomal dominant or X-linked. Alternatively, it may occur in association with Usher's syndrome (deafness and retinitis pigmentosa) or Lawrence-Moon-Biedl syndrome (r. pigmentosa, mental retardation, obesity, hypogonadism and polydactyly).

5 b c e
In papilloedema there is an enlarged blind spot, loss of venous pulsation and constriction of the visual fields but acuity is normal. In papillitis there is diminution of the visual acuity and a central scotoma.

12. Paediatrics

1. **The following developmental milestones would be regarded as normal in a child if it:**
   a. holds head up at 6 months
   b. crawls by 1 year
   c. has pincer grasp at 6 months
   d. sits unaided at 6 months
   e. drinks from cup at 18 months

2. **Fetal infections which are acquired transplacentally include:**
   a. toxoplasmosis
   b. *Escherichia coli*
   c. Herpes hominis
   d. *Neisseria gonorrhoeae*
   e. cytomegalovirus

3. **Regarding respiratory distress syndrome of the newborn:**
   a. it occurs within 1–2 days of birth
   b. lung compliance is increased
   c. babies who survive are more prone to infections later
   d. maternal toxaemia is a predisposing factor
   e. babies tend to be pyrexial

4. **Bronchiolitis in infants:**
   a. is usually a mild respiratory illness
   b. is caused by respiratory syncytial virus
   c. produces hyperinflation of the chest
   d. occurs in summer epidemics
   e. results in loss of cilia from the respiratory membranes

5. **The following are characteristically found in Reye's syndrome:**
   a. hyperglycaemia
   b. lactic acidosis
   c. jaundice
   d. elevated hepatic transaminases
   e. fatty degeneration of the liver

(Answers overleaf)

1 b e
An infant can usually hold its head up by 3 months, attains pincer grasp by 9–12 months and sits unaided by about 9 months.

2 a e
Toxoplasmosis, CMV, rubella and herpes infections are the best known causes of congenital infection. Herpes, Listeria, *E. coli* and *N. gonorrhoeae* cause infection via the birth canal. Syphilitic infection is not seen commonly now but was a known transplacental cause of infection.

3 none
RDS occurs within a few hours of birth and is manifested by an increase in respiratory rate, expiratory grunting and sternal and intercostal recession. Lung compliance and surfactant are decreased and babies who survive are *not* more prone to infection later. Maternal toxaemia and heroin addiction, if anything, protect against development of RDS. Predisposing factors include maternal diabetes mellitus, prematurity and perinatal asphyxia.

4 b c e
Bronchiolitis is most commonly caused by respiratory syncytial virus producing a severe acute infection with outbreaks in winter. It affects mainly infants and toddlers. The respiratory rate rises and babies may present with feeding difficulties, tachycardia, cyanosis, hyperinflation of the chest, widespread crepitations and rhonchi.

5 b d e
Reye's syndrome has been linked to a mild viral infection with influenza virus (A and B) as well as varicella infection. There is fatty degeneration of the liver, high serum ammonia levels, prolonged prothrombin time, hypoglycaemia, raised creatine phosphokinase, lactic acidosis and elevated AST/ALT. Death occurs in 50% cases and jaundice is not a feature.

6 Convulsions in the first week of life can be attributed to:
a hypomagnesaemia
b hypercalcaemia
c metabolic alkalosis
d intrapartum hypoxia
e hyperbilirubinaemia

7 The following are characteristic of babies with pyloric stenosis:
a males are affected more often than females
b symptoms begin in the first week of life
c babies tend to be apathetic and disinterested
d barium meal examination may be diagnostic
e the urine will be alkaline because of repeated vomiting

8 Histiocytosis X:
a may present as pneumothorax
b produces predominantly lower zone infiltrates on chest x-ray
c leads to osteosclerotic skull lesions
d may be diagnosed by broncho-alveolar lavage
e is commonly associated with skin rashes

9 Nephroblastoma:
a shows a predilection for the left kidney
b is associated with aniridia
c may contain striated muscle
d in 10% cases is bilateral
e once diagnosed nephrectomy should be performed as an emergency

10 The following disorders are attributable to defects as described:
a cystinosis is a defect of the proximal tubule resulting in rickets and renal failure
b nephrogenic diabetes insipidus results from reduced sensitivity of the distal tubule to ADH
c Fanconi's syndrome is a generalised tubular defect which may result in rickets
d Hartnup disease results from a generalised tubular defect which results in cerebellar ataxia
e lead poisoning affects predominantly the proximal tubule resulting in anaemia

11 The following produce a transient neonatal hypoparathyroidism:
a cerebral injury
b DiGeorge syndrome
c thymic aplasia
d prematurity
e maternal diabetes

(Answers overleaf)

6 a d e
Convulsions in the first week of life may be caused by infection, hypoglycaemia, intrapartum hypoxia, acidosis, narcotic withdrawal, hypocalcaemia, hypomagnesaemia, hypernatraemia and hyperbilirubinaemia.

7 a d
This condition affects 2/1000 live births and males>females. Symptoms begin 3–6 weeks after birth with projectile vomiting. The vomit is not bile-stained and the baby tends to be constipated. On examination the baby is alert, anxious and hungry. Barium meal examination may be diagnostic showing an elongated and rather narrow pylorus. The urine will be acid (paradoxical acid urine).

8 a d e
Histiocytosis X may present as pneumothorax, otitis media or upper respiratory tract infection. Classical features are diabetes insipidus. exophthalmos and osteolytic skull lesions. Diagnosis may be made by broncho-alveolar lavage.

9 a b c d
The incidence is 1/10 000 live births. The left kidney is affected more often than the right; 10% are bilateral. Nephrectomy should not be delayed but is not regarded as an emergency procedure. The tumour may contain striated and non-striated muscle as well as bone and glandular tissue.

10 b c e
Cystinosis is a generalised renal tubular transport defect resulting in rickets and renal failure. Hartnup disease is a specific transport defect of the proximal tubule leading to pellagra, cerebellar ataxia and mental retardation. Lead poisoning leads to a generalised proximal tubular defect resulting in anaemia and neurological complications.

11 a d e
Transient neonatal hypoparathyroidism may result from cerebral injury, maternal diabetes mellitus, maternal hyperparathyroidism and prematurity. Permanent hypoparathyroidism may be seen in DiGeorge syndrome, autoimmune disease, post-thyroidectomy and aplasia of the thymus.

12 Features consistent with anaphylactoid (Henoch Schönlein) purpura include:
a arthritis affecting mainly small joints
b purpuric rash restricted to buttocks and thighs
c microscopic haematuria
d mild segmental glomerulonephritis
e corticosteroids are often required in the treatment

13 In Prader-Willi syndrome:
a the child's IQ is usually just below normal
b the child has hypotonic limbs
c affected individuals have large hands and feet
d short stature is usual
e affected children are usually obese

14 The following conditions lead to disproportionate short stature:
a hypophosphataemic rickets
b hypothyroidism
c Turner's syndrome
d coeliac disease
e hypophosphatasia

15 In acrodermatitis enteropathica:
a the cause is thought to be magnesium deficiency
b the outcome may be fatal
c alopecia is common
d IgA deficiency occurs
e there is a characteristic rash over the pressure areas

(Answers overleaf)

12 c d
Henoch Schönlein purpura is a diffuse self-limiting condition producing localised oedema of the hands and face. There is a maculopapular rash on the buttocks and extensor surfaces of the legs. Nephritis, abdominal pain, haematemesis, melaena and intussusception are features. The rash is not thrombocytopenic and the condition tends to follow an upper respiratory tract infection in the spring.

13 b d e
The Prader-Willi syndrome is characterised by an IQ of 40–60, short stature, hypotonia, small hands/feet and hypogonadism.

14 a e
Proportionate short stature is a feature of Turner's syndrome, hypothyroidism and coeliac disease. Disproportionate short stature is seen in hypophosphataemic rickets, hypophosphatasia and achondroplasia.

15 b c e
This disorder is linked to an abnormality of zinc metabolism. Babies develop severe diarrhoea and failure to thrive is common. The rash is most prominent at mucocutaneous junctions and over pressure areas. Alopecia and dystrophy of the nails are recognised. If untreated it may be fatal.

13. Pharmacology

1. **The following antibiotics in therapeutic dosage are bactericidal:**
   a. penicillins
   b. erythromycin
   c. tetracyclines
   d. aminoglycosides
   e. cephalosporins

2. **The following are recognised effects of atropine:**
   a. hyperthermia
   b. bronchial smooth muscle relaxation
   c. sweating
   d. increased smooth muscle tone in the gut
   e. increased intra-ocular pressure

3. **Interactions recognised as dangerous occurs between mono-amine oxidase inhibitors and:**
   a. yeast
   b. chlorpheniramine
   c. aspirin
   c. L-dopa
   e. pethidine

4. **Recognised side effects of phenytoin include:**
   a. osteoporosis
   b. folate deficiency
   c. nystagmus
   d. hirsutism
   e. fever

5. **Shortening of the QT interval on the ECG is a feature of:**
   a. quinidine treatment
   b. administration of amiodarone
   c. digoxin toxicity
   d. hypercalcaemia
   e. phenothiazine treatment

(Answers overleaf)

1 a d e
Bacteriostatic drugs include: tetracyclines, trimethoprim, sulphonamides, lincomycin and chloramphenicol. Bactericidal agents include the aminoglycosides, penicillins, cotrimoxazole and isoniazid.

2 a b e
Atropine blocks muscarinic cholinergic receptors and is used widely as a premedication because of its ability to dry up secretions. Its side effects include tachycardia, pupillary dilatation, reduced sweating, pyrexia and reduced muscle tone in bladder and uterus.

3 a b d e
Mono-amine oxidase inhibitors (MAOIs) inhibit mitochondrial mono-amine oxidases resulting in increased stores of 5-hydroxytryptamine, noradrenaline and dopamine. Interactions occur between MAOIs and amphetamines, L-dopa, barbiturates and tricyclics. Foods which may be dangerous if taken in combination with MAOIs include Bovril, Marmite, Chianti wine, cheese and green figs.

4 b c d e
Phenytoin has many side effects including rashes, fever, hepatitis, SLE, gingival hyperplasia, thickened facial tissues, acne, lymphadenopathy, cerebellar syndrome and sedation.

5 c d
The QT interval varies with age and heart rate (reduced in tachycardia and increased in bradycardia). The QT interval is shortened in pyrexia, digoxin toxicity, hypercalcaemia and with vagal stimulation. Quinidine, tricyclics, amiodarone, hypocalcaemia and increased intracranial pressure lead to prolongation of the QT interval.

PHARMACOLOGY

6 The following drug combinations may produce unwanted effects:
  a metformin and cimetidine
  b digoxin and amiodarone
  c calcium salts and thiazides
  d thyroxine and frusemide
  e acetazolamide and aspirin

7 The following agents are recognised bronchoconstrictors:
  a kinins
  b atropine
  c prostaglandin E
  d 5-hydroxytryptamine
  e prostaglandin F2α

8 The following statements concerning cimetidine are true:
  a potentiation of aminophylline may occur
  b metabolism of propranolol is enhanced
  c gynaecomastia but not hyperprolactinaemia are recognised
  d cimetidine is ineffective in blocking acid secretion in response to caffeine
  e confusion in the elderly which rapidly responds to withdrawal of the drug has been described

9 Loop diuretics have been shown to:
  a cause neutropenia
  b induce hyperchloraemic alkalosis
  c induce thrombocytopenia
  d interfere with countercurrent exchange in the kidney
  e cause muscle pain in some cases

10 The urine becomes acid if the following agents are administered:
  a oral arginine
  b intravenous lactate
  c oral ascorbic acid
  d oral methionine
  e oral citrate

11 The following are true of oral contraceptives:
  a there is a decreased risk of ovarian carcinoma
  b suppression of benign breast disease is recognised
  c there is a decreased risk of cervical erosion
  d breakthrough bleeding may occur with concomitant administration of griseofulvin
  e hepatocellular adenoma is a risk

(Answers overleaf)

6 a b c e
Metformin given with cimetidine may result in increased concentrations of the former. Digoxin given with amiodarone or quinine results in digoxin potentiation and the dose should be reduced. With thiazides, caution should be exercised when using calcium salts because of the increased risk of hypercalcaemia. Acetazolamide given with aspirin results in reduced excretion of the acetazolamide and hence increased risk of toxicity.

7 a d e
Agents shown to act as bronchoconstrictors include kinins, prostaglandin (PG)F2α, histamine, acetylcholine, SRSA, 5HT and β blockers (in asthmatics). Bronchodilators are: β agonists, theophylline, atropine and PGE.

8 a e
Cimetidine is a competitive H2 antagonist. It blocks nocturnal and basal acid secretion and also blocks acid secretion in response to food, insulin and caffeine. Adverse effects include diarrhoea, rashes, dizziness, gynaecomastia and hyperprolactinaemia.

9 a c d e
Loop diuretics are: frusemide, bumetanide and ethacrynic acid. They are absorbed rapidly from the gut and side effects include hypokalaemia, hypovolaemia, impaired glucose tolerance, uric acid retention, nephrotoxicity and ototoxicity. Bumetanide occasionally causes muscle pain.

10 a c d
Compounds which make the urine acid include oral ammonium chloride, oral methionine, oral arginine and oral ascorbic acid. The urine becomes alkaline if IV lactate, IV/oral sodium bicarbonate or oral Na^+/K^+ citrate are administered.

11 a b d e
Oestrogens act as contraceptive agents by inhibiting gonadotrophin release and progestogens act by modifying cervical mucus preventing implantation of the zygote.
Advantages conferred by the oestrogen-containing contraceptives are: reduced frequency of benign breast disease, reduced incidence of ovarian cysts and control of functional uterine bleeding. However, cervical erosions are more likely and hepatocellular adenoma is recognised. Thrombo-embolic disease is increased.

PHARMACOLOGY

12 The following statements are true of growth hormone:
  a levels increase during hypoglycaemia
  b decreased levels are detected during slow wave sleep
  c somatomedin secretion by the liver is stimulated
  d levels are independent of protein consumption
  e the molecular weight is about 2000

13 Agents which decrease thyroid binding globulin concentration include:
  a viral hepatitis
  b nephrotic syndrome
  c oestrogens
  d phenytoin
  e phenothiazines

14 Substances known to stimulate insulin release include:
  a gastrin
  b cAMP
  c diazoxide
  d α-agonists
  e thyroxine

15 Potentiation of warfarin occurs with:
  a liquid paraffin
  b griseofulvin
  c clofibrate
  d phenytoin
  e chlorpropamide

16 Anticancer agents which act on the 'S' phase of the cell cycle include:
  a vincristine
  b actinomycin D
  c asparaginase
  d 6-mercaptopurine
  e methotrexate

17 Hirsutism is a recognised side effect of:
  a progestogens
  b guanethidine
  c psoralens
  d ethacrynic acid
  e trimethoprim

(Answers overleaf)

12 a c
Growth hormone is produced by the pituitary gland. Levels increase in patients on L-dopa, during slow wave sleep, during hypoglycaemia and stress. Levels are decreased in patients on corticosteroids, with the administration of glucose and after ingestion of protein. Bromocriptine, a dopamine agonist, is used to block production of growth hormone in cases where serum levels are raised.

13 b d
Thyroid binding globulin (TBG) levels are decreased in patients on corticosteroids, androgens and phenytoin and in nephrotic syndrome. An increase in TBG may be seen with administration of oestrogens, clofibrate, phenothiazines, viral hepatitis and myxoedema.

14 a b e
Insulin release is stimulated by a variety of factors including carbohydrate ingestion, free fatty acids, glucagon, growth hormone, oestrogens and thyroxine. Secretion is inhibited by β blockers, α agonists and diazoxide.

15 a c e
Warfarin prevents the synthesis of the vitamin K-dependent clotting factors (II, VII, IX and X). Potentiation may occur with non-steroidal anti-inflammatory drugs, nalidixic acid, alcohol, cholestyramine, amiodarone, cimetidine and broad-spectrum antibiotics.

16 b c d e
'S' phase corresponds to the phase in the cell cycle in which DNA synthesis takes place. Some drugs (alkylating agents) act on all phases whereas others are phase-specific, acting on one particular phase in the cycle. Actinomycin D, asparaginase, 6-mercaptopurine, 5-fluorouracil and cytosine arabinoside are phase-specific and act on 'S' phase.

17 a c
Those drugs which may induce hirsutism include phenytoin, minoxidil (now used in the treatment of baldness), anabolic steroids, progestogens and diazoxide.

18 Drugs which are safe in pregnancy include:
  a frusemide
  b ethambutol
  c cephalosporins
  d hydralazine
  e reserpine

19 Drugs which can be given safely to breast-feeding mothers include:
  a warfarin
  b amiodarone
  c bromides
  d carbamazepine
  e carbimazole

20 The following drugs are recognised goitrogens:
  a cholestyramine
  b warfarin
  c phenylbutazone
  d para-amino salicylic acid
  e lithium

21 The following drugs should not be given to patients with renal failure:
  a vancomycin
  b ethambutol
  c demeclocycline
  d griseofulvin
  e rifampicin

22 Cigarette smokers may require higher doses than non-smokers of:
  a phenytoin
  b diazepam
  c imipramine
  d theophylline
  e chlorpromazine

23 The following drugs should be avoided in patients with porphyria:
  a griseofulvin
  b aspirin
  c pethidine
  d thiopentone
  e penicillin

(Answers overleaf)

18 b c d
Frusemide causes a reduction in plasma volume and thereby reduces placental perfusion and should not be used in the treatment of hypertension in pregnancy. Reserpine causes neonatal bradycardia and drowsiness and should be avoided in pregnancy.

19 a d
Drugs excreted in breast milk and which may affect the baby include choramphenicol, amiodarone, barbiturates, lithium, aspirin and ergotamine.

20 c d e
Other drugs which may induce goitre are iodides and sulphonamides.

21 a b
Vancomycin should not be given intravenously if possible. Ethambutol is best avoided if the GFR<50 ml/min. The others are probably safe. Other agents to avoid are nalidixic acid, tetracyclines (apart from demeclocycline) and nitrofurantoin.

22 c d e
Smoking accelerates the metabolism of paracetamol, imipramine, phenobarbitone, caffeine and theophylline and smokers may need higher doses to have the same effects as non-smokers. Phenytoin, alcohol and diazepam are unaffected by smoking.

23 a d
Drugs safe to use in acute porphyria include pethidine, chlorpromazine, aspirin, penicillin and diazepam. Those to be avoided are barbiturates, glutethimide, phenytoin, alcohol, sulphonamides, sex hormones and methyldopa.

24 The following statements are true:
  a phenacetin-induced methaemoglobinaemia is inherited as an autosomal dominant
  b malignant hyperpyrexia is seen only with halothane
  c patients with Down's syndrome are more sensitive than normal to anticholinergic agents
  d Gilbert's disease may be exacerbated by oestrogens
  e acatalasia predisposes to oral and pharyngeal infection

25 Drugs which are eliminated by rendering the urine alkaline include:
  a amphetamine
  b phenobarbitone
  c pethidine
  d barbitone
  e aspirin

(Answers overleaf)

24 c d e
Phenacetin-induced methaemoglobinaemia is inherited as an autosomal recessive. The condition is due to a defect in mixed function de-ethylating activity in the liver leading to methaemoglobinaemia with phenacetin ingestion. Malignant hyperpyrexia may be seen with a variety of anaesthetic agents including halothane and suxamethonium. Inheritance is autosomal dominant. Gilbert's disease (familial unconjugated hyperbilirubinaemia) is treated prophylactically with barbiturates and made worse by oestrogens and starvation. Acatalasia is a condition in which the red blood cell catalase is defective and is inherited as an autosomal recessive.

25 b d e
Alkaline diuresis may be used to eliminate salicylates. phenobarbitone and barbitone. These drugs are maximally ionised in an alkaline environment and tubular reabsorption is reduced and excretion is therefore enhanced.

14. Renal disease

1. **The following are true of antidiuretic hormone (ADH) release:**
   a. ADH is released in response to rising plasma osmolality
   b. hypokalaemia leads to a reduction in its effects on the collecting ducts
   c. ADH activates adenyl cyclase
   d. the serum osmolality threshold for ADH release is 280 mosm/kg
   e. in the absence of ADH release urine flow is 40l/24 hours

2. **Papillary necrosis can be attributed to:**
   a. sickle cell anaemia
   b. diabetes mellitus
   c. renal TB
   d. paracetamol
   e. glucose-6-phosphate dehydrogenase deficiency

3. **The following stones are radiolucent:**
   a. silicate
   b. cystine
   c. uric acid
   d. xanthine
   e. ammonium phosphate

4. **Causes of a large kidney include:**
   a. nephrotic syndrome
   b. renal artery stenosis
   c. compulsive beer drinking
   d. hypernephroma
   e. chronic glomerulonephritis

5. **The following are found in renal tubular acidosis:**
   a. hypouricaemia
   b. hyperkalaemia
   c. bone pain
   d. high serum bicarbonate
   e. high urine pH

(Answers overleaf)

1 a b c d
ADH is released from the posterior pituitary in response to low cardiac output, dehydration, pain and an increase in plasma osmolality (threshold 280 mosmol/kg). It binds to the collecting duct basement membrane and activates adenyl cyclase leading to cAMP production. With ADH release the urine output may drop to 500 ml/24 hours or rise to 20l/24 hours in its absence.

2 a b c
Renal papillary necrosis is classically associated with analgesic abuse (e.g. phenacetin) and is thought to be due to concentration of the offending drug in the renal pyramids leading to ischaemia and necrosis. Patients may present with renal failure, hypertension, renal colic, haematuria or distal renal tubular acidosis (RTA). The condition predisposes to carcinoma of the renal pelvis. The condition is also associated with sickle cell anaemia, diabetes mellitus, renal tuberculosis and macroglobulinaemia.

3 c d
Uric acid and xanthine stones are radiolucent. Calcium, magnesium, cystine, silicate and struvite stones are radio-opaque.

4 a c d
The kidney is normally between 11 and 14 cm long. Unilateral large kidneys are seen in renal vein thrombosis, duplex kidney and hypernephroma. Bilateral enlargement is a feature of the nephrotic syndrome, acute renal failure, acute pyelonephritis, polycystic kidneys and acromegaly.

5 a c e
See 'Metabolic Disease' Qu. 3.

The urine will show hypercalciuria, low specific gravity, pH>6.0 and decreased ammonium. There will be hyperchloraemia, hypokalaemia, low serum bicarbonate, low serum uric acid and phosphate. The anion gap will be normal.

RENAL DISEASE

6 The following indicate a poor prognosis in the nephrotic syndrome:
- a hypercholesterolaemia
- b hypertension
- c low serum complement levels
- d hypo-albuminaemia
- e non-selective proteinuria

7 Diseases in which complement levels are normal include:
- a systemic lupus erythematosus
- b membranous glomerulonephritis
- c IgA nephropathy
- d Goodpasture's syndrome
- e polyarteritis nodosa

8 Haemodialysis may not improve the following features of renal failure:
- a anaemia
- b fluid overload
- c pericarditis
- d hypoalbuminaemia
- e pruritus

9 The finding of a raised anion gap is compatible with:
- a bromism
- b uraemia
- c salicylate poisoning
- d carbenicillin therapy
- e diarrhoea

10 The following endocrine disturbances are recognised in chronic renal failure:
- a hypoglucagonaemia
- b hypergastrinaemia
- c hyperreninaemia
- d diminished fertility
- e hyperparathyroidism

11 The following lead to pyuria:
- a potassium depletion
- b ureteritis cystica
- c probenecid
- d lead poisoning
- e analgesic abuse

(Answers overleaf)

6 b c e
The prognosis is made worse if the GFR<10 ml/min, if there is oliguria, haematuria, non-selective proteinuria, low complement or purpura.

7 b c d e
Complement levels are low in lupus nephritis, acute post-streptococcal nephritis, membranoproliferative glomerulonephritis, bacterial endocarditis, SLE and cryoglobulinaemia. Complement levels are normal in minimal change nephropathy, IgA nephropathy, Goodpasture's syndrome, polyarteritis nodosa and Wegener's granulomatosis.

8 a c e
Haemodialysis may not improve pericarditis, renal bone disease, anaemia, itch, neuropathy and the increased risk of cardiovascular disease. Indications for dialysis include diuretic-resistant overload, resistant hypertension, hyperkalaemia and pericarditis.

9 b c d
The anion gap ('Metabolic Disease' Qu. 16) is normally 8–12. An increased anion gap is seen in lactic acidosis, diabetic keto-acidosis, alcoholic ketoacidosis, methanol and ethylene glycol poisoning, starvation, salicylate overdose and renal failure. The anion gap is normal in diarrhoea, RTA (distal and proximal), ureterosigmoidostomy, pancreatic losses and in patients on acetazolamide.

10 b c d e
In chronic renal failure there may be hypocalcaemia, hypo-albuminaemia and low serum zinc levels. Metabolic acidosis, hyperkalaemia, hyperphosphataemia, hyperuricaemia, hypermagnesaemia and hyperreninaemia are features. Gastrin and glucagon levels may be elevated and secondary hyperparathyroidism is characteristic.

11 a b d e
Pyuria may be a consequence of analgesic abuse, lead poisoning, potassium depletion, nephrocalcinosis, medullary sponge kidney and radiation nephritis. Infections of the urinary tract as well as acute/chronic interstitial nephritis also lead to pyuria.

RENAL DISEASE

12 The following cause the urine to turn red:
   a amitriptyline
   b phenolphthalein in alkaline urine
   c methaemoglobin
   d myoglobinuria
   e desferrioxamine

13 Findings consistent with a diagnosis of retroperitoneal fibrosis include:
   a raised ESR
   b heart block
   c loin pain
   d portal hypertension
   e weight loss

14 Conditions associated with low renin levels include:
   a haemorrhage
   b Conn's syndrome
   c β blockade
   d Cushing's syndrome
   e pregnancy

15 ECG manifestations of hypokalaemia include:
   a prolongation of the PR interval
   b widening of the QRS complex
   c large P wave
   d ST depression
   e prolongation of the QT interval

16 The following drugs induce hyponatraemia:
   a vincristine
   b cyclophosphamide
   c lithium
   d carbamazepine
   e morphine

17 The conditions below produce a strongly acid urine:
   a pyloric stenosis
   b chronic obstructive airways disease
   c renal tubular acidosis
   d chronic renal failure
   e *Proteus* infection

(Answers overleaf)

12   b d e
Urine may turn red with the administration of rifampicin and desferrioxamine. The presence of haemoglobin or myoglobin in the urine will cause a similar urine colour. In alkaptonuria (homogentisic acid in the urine) as well as methaemoglobinuria a blue-black urine may be seen.

13   a b c d e
This condition is associated with treatment with methysergide, ergot alkaloids, hydralazine, sclerosing cholangitis and retroperitoneal lymphomas. Patients may present with weight loss, hypertension and urinary symptoms. Complications include portal hypertension, pulmonary fibrosis, ureteric obstruction and heart block.

14   b c d
Renin is a protease of molecular weight 40 000 produced by the juxtaglomerular apparatus. It catalyses the hydrolysis of angiotensinogen to angiotensin I leading to vasoconstriction. Elevated levels may be seen in Addison's disease, haemorrhage, pregnancy and patients on treatment with diuretics and lithium. Levels may be raised in malignant and some cases of essential hypertension. Low renin levels are associated with most cases of essential hypertension, old age, β blockade and patients on steroids. Renin levels are lower in the supine than standing position.

15   a d e
In hypokalaemia the ECG may show prolonged QT interval, prolonged PR interval, ST depression and T inversion. 'U' waves are more prominent. In hyperkalaemia the T waves are large and tented, the PR interval is prolonged, P waves are flattened and QRS complexes are wide.

16   a b d e
Hyponatraemia may be due to chlorpropamide, thiazides, morphine, carbamazepine, vincristine and cyclophosphamide. Non-drug causes include excess water intake, inappropriate antidiuretic hormone secretion, vomiting, diarrhoea and Addison's disease.

17   a b d
Proteus urinary tract infection and RTA are associated with urine which is alkaline. Pyloric stenosis, COAD and chronic renal failure produce an acid urine.

RENAL DISEASE

18 Alport's syndrome:
   a is inherited as an autosomal recessive
   b leads to optic atrophy
   c has a worse prognosis in males
   d may result in sensorineural deafness
   e can be diagnosed antenatally

19 Prerenal uraemia may be distinguished from established acute tubular necrosis (ATN) by the following:
   a in prerenal uraemia the urine Na^+ is >20 mEq/l
   b in ATN there may be granular casts
   c in ATN the urine:plasma creatinine concentration is <15
   d in prerenal uraemia urine osmolality is >500 mosm/l
   e patients with ATN have a urine:plasma osmolality of >1:1

20 The following genetic diseases are correctly matched with renal abnormalities which may occur:
   a Marfan's syndrome — ectopic kidneys
   b familial Mediterranean fever — nephrocalcinosis
   c hemihypertrophy — nephroblastoma
   d Lawrence-Moon-Biedl syndrome — renal hypoplasia
   e Turner's syndrome — obstructive uropathy

(Answers overleaf)

18 c d
Alport's disease is inherited as an autosomal dominant (variable penetrance/expressivity) associated with nephritis, deafness and lens abnormalities. The condition tends to be worse in males and does not recur after transplantation.

19 b c d
In ATN the urine Na^+ is >20 mEq/l, urine osmolality <400 mosm/l, urine:plasma osmolality is 0.9–1.05 and urine:plasma creatinine concentration is <15. In prerenal uraemia the urine Na^+ is <10 mEq/l, urine osmolality is >500 mosm/l, urine:plasma osmolality >1:1 and urine:plasma creatinine concentration is >20.

20 a c d
Marfan's syndrome is associated with ectopic kidneys, lens dislocation and arachnodactyly. Familial Mediterranean fever is associated with renal amyloid, fever, polyserositis and synovitis. Nephroblastoma may occur in hemihypertrophy and horseshoe kidney/cystic dysplasia are features of Turner's syndrome. Lawrence-Moon-Biedl syndrome is associated with renal hypoplasia, lower renal tract obstruction, polydactyly and mental retardation.

15. Respiratory medicine

1 **Conditions which produce predominantly basal changes on the chest x-ray include:**
   a fibrosing alveolitis
   b aspergillosis
   c sarcoidosis
   d bronchiectasis
   e scleroderma

2 **The following dusts are fibrogenic:**
   a beryllium
   b titanium
   c silica
   d cobalt
   e chromite

3 **In Kartagener's syndrome:**
   a paranasal sinusitis is a feature
   b inheritance is autosomal recessive
   c the underlying pathology lies in collagen structure
   d bronchiectasis is a feature
   e sperm are immotile

4 **The following are true of coalworker's pneumoconiosis:**
   a there is an increased risk of lung cancer
   b particles of 0.5–7.0 μm are most likely to be deposited and engulfed by macrophages
   c the condition frequently causes no symptoms or signs
   d progressive massive fibrosis produces a mixed restrictive and obstructive ventilatory defect
   e the risk of developing tuberculosis is increased

(Answers overleaf)

1 a d e
Basal chest x-ray changes are seen in bronchiectasis, asbestosis, aspiration, pulmonary haemosiderosis, extrinsic allergic alveolitis and idiopathic pulmonary fibrosis. Aspergillosis (if allergic) produces transient CXR shadows; aspergilloma affects the upper lobes. Sarcoidosis produces miliary mottling, ground-glass appearance and honeycomb lung.

2 a c d
Beryllium, cobalt, mercury, asbestos, kaolin and silica are fibrogenic. Titanium and chromite are non-fibrogenic. Granulomas occur with talc, beryllium and aluminium.

3 a b d e
Kartagener's syndrome is associated with sinusitis, bronchiectasis, absent frontal sinuses, dextrocardia and immotile sperm. The condition is caused by ciliary abnormalities and affected males are infertile.

4 b c d
In simple pneumoconiosis the CXR shows widespread 1–2 mm opacities. The condition is asymptomatic until progressive massive fibrosis (PMF) occurs. Simple pneumoconiosis does not progress if exposure is stopped, whereas PMF does. There is no increase in the risk of developing lung cancer. There is, however, an increased risk of developing pulmonary tuberculosis in pneumoconiosis produced by silica but not PMF.

5 Findings in a patient with fibrosing alveolitis include:
   a an obstructive ventilatory defect
   b reduced transfer factor
   c normal pCO_2 and pO_2
   d hypertrophic pulmonary osteoarthropathy
   e increased lung compliance

6 The following drugs produce eosinophilic alveolar reactions:
   a sulphasalazine
   b nitrofurantoin
   c chlorambucil
   d carbamazepine
   e amiodarone

7 Alveolar-capillary block is attributable to the following:
   a post-lung resection
   b pneumonia
   c chronic bronchitis
   d asbestosis
   e asthma

8 Pulmonary alveolar proteinosis:
   a is associated with hilar lymphadenopathy
   b predisposes to *Nocardia* infection
   c is more common in females
   d produces an obstructive ventilatory defect
   e can be monitored by serial lactate dehydrogenase (LDH) measurements

9 The following statements about carbon monoxide poisoning are true:
   a the O_2 dissociation curve is shifted to the right
   b cerebral oedema occurs
   c the half-life of elimination of carbon monoxide from the blood is about 50 minutes when the patient breathes 100% O_2
   d the oxygen tension is normal
   e alveolar ventilation is reduced

(Answers overleaf)

5 b c d
This results in interstitial pulmonary fibrosis and may be an isolated finding or is sometimes found in conjunction with a connective tissue disorder (rheumatoid arthritis, SLE, scleroderma, coeliac disease, renal tubular acidosis or dermatomyositis). There is progressive exertional dyspnoea, dry cough, gross clubbing and numerous late-inspiratory crepitations. Lung function tests show a restrictive ventilatory defect, reduced TL_{co} and decreased lung compliance. Blood testing may show positive rheumatoid factor, antinuclear factor, raised ESR and elevated gamma globulins.

6 a b d
Pulmonary eosinophilia may result from the administration of nitrofurantoin, aspirin, chlorpropamide, sulphasalazine, imipramine and phenylbutazone. Infections such as *Ascaris lumbricoides*, microfilaria and *Aspergillus fumigatus* may also lead to pulmonary eosinophilia.

7 a b d
Alveolar-capillary block results from widespread thickening of the alveolar walls. This is associated with fibrosing alveolitis, post-lung resection, extensive fibrosis, emphysema, lymphangitis carcinomatosa, pneumonia and scleroderma. Chronic bronchitis and asthma are not causes of alveolar-capillary block.

8 b d e
The aetiology of this condition is unknown. It affects M>F in the 20–55 year age group. The alveoli fill with PAS-positive proteinaceous material. The onset is insidious and patients expectorate mucoid sputum. Clubbing is a feature. Diagnosis is made by lung biopsy and LDH measurements may be used to monitor treatment. Treatment is largely by bronchoalveolar lavage. Steroids have no role in treatment.

9 b c d
$CO + Hb$ = carboxyhaemoglobin. The total O_2 carrying capacity drops and the O_2 dissociation curve shifts to the *Left*. Arterial O_2 saturation is decreased but O_2 tension is normal. The half-life of elimination of CO in 100% O_2 is 50 minutes and ≈22 minutes in hyperbaric oxygen.

10 Pneumothorax is associated with:
a hydatid cyst
b tuberose sclerosis
c endometriosis
d Ehlers Danlos syndrome
e silicosis

11 Theophylline clearance is reduced in:
a patients with fever
b acute viral infection
c children
d heart failure
e patients receiving cimetidine

12 The following are true of restrictive lung disease:
a the vital capacity is increased
b total lung capacity is decreased
c FEV_1:FVC ratio is greater than 70%
d pleural effusion may be a cause
e residual volume is increased

13 Obstructive sleep apnoea is associated with:
a nocturnal enuresis
b hyperthyroidism
c superior vena cava obstruction
d acromegaly
e intellectual impairment

14 The following produce anterior mediastinal masses
a dermoid cyst
b ganglioneuroma
c teratoma
d thymoma
e Zenker's diverticulum

15 Good prognostic indicators in sarcoidosis include:
a HLA B8
b acute uveitis
c strongly-positive gallium scan
d heavy lymphocytosis on bronchoalveolar lavage
e erythema nodosum

16 Pleural effusions:
a tend to be transudates in Meig's syndrome
b are chylous in lymphoma
c with elevated amylase are diagnostic of acute pancreatitis
d have a high glucose content in rheumatoid arthritis
e have a low pH in oesophageal rupture

(Answers overleaf)

10 a b c d e
Pneumothorax is associated with a variety of conditions including idiopathic (majority), COAD with rupture of bullae, staphylococcal lung abscess, pulmonary infarction, bronchial carcinoma, asthma, rib fracture, cystic fibrosis, berylliosis, Ehlers Danlos syndrome, Marfan's syndrome and endometriosis.

11 a b d e
Theophylline clearance is increased in cigarette smokers, alcoholics and children. Clearance is decreased in liver/heart failure, fever, the elderly, acute viral infections and in patients taking erythromycin.

12 b c d
In restrictive lung disease there is reduction in residual volume, vital capacity and total lung capacity. The $FEV_1:FVC$ ratio may be normal or increased. In obstructive lung disease the residual volume is increased, $FEV_1:FVC$ ratio is decreased and the vital capacity is decreased.

13 a c d e
Obstructive sleep apnoea is associated with hypothyroidism, acromegaly, obesity, tonsillar/adenoid enlargement and SVC obstruction. The patient snores loudly, is sleepy during the day and may suffer impairment of the intellect. Personality change and nocturnal enuresis are features. The *obstructive* form is commoner than the *central* type, the latter being associated with normal body size, light snoring and depression.

14 a c d
Anterior mediastinal masses may be seen with retrosternal goitre, thymomas, lymphomas, teratomas and aortic aneurysm. Zenker's diverticulum (hypopharyngeal diverticulum) is found in the superior mediastinum and ganglioneuromas are found in the posterior mediastinum.

15 a b e
Good prognostic indicators are: bilateral hilar lymphadenopathy, F>M, HLA B8, erythema nodosum, acute uveitis and arthritis. A strongly-positive gallium scan and heavy lymphocytosis on bronchoalveolar lavage indicate a worse prognosis.

16 a b e
An elevated amylase in a pleural effusion may be found in perforation of the oesophagus and pancreatitis. Rheumatoid arthritis is associated with a *low* glucose. This is also the case in empyema.

17 In α_1-antitrypsin deficiency:
  a inheritance is autosomal dominant
  b a single base change is the underlying defect
  c chest x-ray shows basal hyperlucency
  d emphysema is of a panacinar type
  e mesangiocapillary glomerulonephritis is rarely associated

18 The following are true of Goodpasture's syndrome:
  a circulating immune complexes are found
  b it represents a type II hypersensitivity reaction
  c lesions recur in transplanted kidneys
  d the course is usually rapidly progressive
  e the associated glomerulonephritis is usually mild

19 Concerning bronchoalveolar lavage (BAL):
  a the FEV_1 must be greater than 2l before attempting the procedure
  b BAL may help in the diagnosis of occupational lung diseases
  c the lavage fluid contains Langerhan's cells in patients with histiocytosis X
  d the number of macrophages in lavage fluid is decreased in patients who are cigarette smokers
  e the technique provides a form of therapy for alveolar proteinosis

20 Sarcoidosis is associated with:
  a elevated transfer factor
  b ocular pain
  c nephrocalcinosis
  d enlarged paratracheal lymph nodes
  e small airways obstruction

(Answers overleaf)

17 b c d e
In α_1-antitrypsin deficiency there is an absent α_1 band on protein electrophoresis. It may lead to liver disease in childhood and cirrhosis/emphysema in adults. Inheritance is autosomal recessive and produces a severe panacinar emphysema affecting the lower lobes predominantly.

18 b c d
Glomerulonephritis (severe) and intra-alveolar haemorrhage occur. CXR shows generalised mottling. There is no arteritis and there are *no* circulating immune complexes. Without treatment the mean survival is 15 weeks.

19 b c d e
This technique is useful for monitoring disease progress in sarcoidosis, fibrosing alveolitis, extrinsic allergic alveolitis and histiocytosis X. It may also provide a form of therapy for pulmonary alveolar proteinosis and sputum retention.

20 b c d e
TL_{co} is decreased, ocular pain occurs due to uveitis, calcium metabolism is deranged resulting in hypercalcaemia, hypercalciuria and nephrocalcinosis.

16. Rheumatology/immunology

1 **Causes of cryoglobulinaemia include:**
   a ulcerative colitis
   b infectious mononucleosis
   c multiple myeloma
   d syphilis
   e systemic lupus erythematosus

2 **A patient is more likely to be suffering from Reiter's disease than Behçet's if:**
   a mouth ulcers are painless
   b the main eye complication is uveitis
   c the patient is HLA B12-positive
   d the patient is male
   e mutilating joint disease is present

3 **The following indicate a poor prognosis in rheumatoid arthritis:**
   a sudden onset
   b eosinophilia
   c cryoglobulinaemia
   d mono-articular presentation
   e very high ESR

4 **D-penicillamine has the following recognised side effects:**
   a myasthenia gravis
   b taste loss
   c convulsions
   d polymyositis
   e ataxia

5 **The following conditions lead to gout in childhood:**
   a hypertriglyceridaemia
   b Von Gierke's disease
   c lead poisoning
   d hypothyroidism
   e sickle cell disease

(Answers overleaf)

1 a b c d e
Symptoms/signs are due to immunoglobulin precipitation at temperatures lower than body temperature and include Raynaud's phenomenon, arthralgia, purpura and renal failure. Causes include infectious mononucleosis, leprosy, SBE, malaria, SLE, rheumatoid arthritis, lymphoma and leukaemia.

2 a d e
Mouth ulcers in Reiter's syndrome are painless but in Behçet's syndrome are painful. The ocular complication of Reiter's is mainly conjunctivitis; uveitis is a feature of Behçet's. HLA B27 is associated with Reiter's and HLA B12 and B5 are found in Behçet's. There is a stronger male preponderance in Reiter's than Behçet's and mutilating joint disease is a feature of Reiter's.

3 b c e
Bad prognostic features include significant weight loss, polyarticular presentation, fever, nodules, pulmonary fibrosis, neurological complications, lymphadenopathy, amyloid, anaemia, hypoalbuminaemia, high ESR, high titre of rheumatoid factor and cryoglobulinaemia.

4 a b d
Penicillamine may cause taste loss and anorexia. Proteinuria and nephrotic syndrome may occur. Rashes, SLE, myasthenia gravis, polymyositis and a Goodpasture-like syndrome are recognised.

5 a b c e
Childhood gout is associated with Lesch-Nyhan syndrome, leukaemia, uncontrolled diabetes mellitus, Von Gierke's disease, Gaucher's disease, lead poisoning and sickle cell disease.

6 In systemic sclerosis:
a males and females are affected in roughly equal frequency
b vitiligo is associated
c half the patients with oesophageal involvement are asymptomatic
d anaemia, when present, is most commonly due to autoimmune haemolysis
e D-penicillamine has been shown to be of benefit in the treatment of visceral involvement

7 In relapsing polychondritis:
a swollen ears are a feature
b saddle nose occurs
c aortic stenosis is associated
d there is a recognised association with other autoimmune diseases
e mortality is low

8 Pleural effusions in rheumatoid arthritis usually show:
a blood staining
b high protein content
c high levels of lactate dehydrogenase
d high C3 complement levels
e immune complexes

9 The following viral infections lead to acute polyarthritis:
a mumps
b human parvovirus
c cytomegalovirus
d influenza
e chickenpox

10 In Fabry's disease:
a inheritance is autosomal dominant
b glycolipids accumulate in synovium
c β-galactosidase deficiency is the underlying defect
d burning joint pain without swelling occurs
e progressive cerebral involvement is the usual cause of death

11 Rheumatological drugs to be avoided in breast-feeding mothers include:
a ibuprofen
b gold
c naproxen
d penicillamine
e flufenamic acid

(Answers overleaf)

6 b c
Systemic sclerosis is a connective tissue disorder which may be generalised or may primarily affect the skin. Females are affected more frequently than males. The condition leads to cardiac, pulmonary, renal, gastrointestinal and haematological complications. The aetiology is unknown and the 5-year survival for progressive systemic sclerosis is about 50%. Oesophageal involvement occurs in the majority of cases but is symptomatic in only half of those affected. Renal disease is associated with hypertension and is a bad prognostic sign. Anaemia is a feature but an autoimmune basis is present in the minority. D-penicillamine may help skin lesions but is of little value in the treatment of visceral involvement.

7 a b d
This condition affects the mucopolysaccharide component of cartilage. This leads to inflammation and weakening of cartilage of the ear, nose, larynx and trachea. It is associated with rheumatoid arthritis, SLE, Sjögren's syndrome, ulcerative colitis and diabetes mellitus. Mortality is not low and death may be due to rupture of an aortic aneurysm or pneumonia.

8 b c e
Pleural effusions in rheumatoid arthritis have high protein and lactate dehydrogenase levels, low sugar and C3 and are positive for rheumatoid factor. The fluid may be turbid due to the presence of white blood cells but should not be blood-stained.

9 b c d
Hepatitis B and A, can produce polyarthritis. In infection with human parvovirus there may also be erythema infectiosum (slapped cheek syndrome). Other causes of polyarthritis include infection with *Staphylococcus aureus, Salmonella, Neisseria gonorrhoeae* and *Mycoplasma* as well as Lyme disease, rubella and brucellosis.

10 b d e
This is a rare sex-linked condition in which there is widespread accumulation of glycolipid in brain, kidney, lens and synovium. The deficiency is of α-galactosidase. Severe burning joint pain and angiokeratoma are features. No treatment is available at present.

11 b d
Gold is excreted in breast milk and may produce rashes in the breast-feeding baby.

12 The following statements about the complement system are true:
    a   IgM and IgG are responsible for activating the classical pathway
    b   C2 induces vascular permeability
    c   C3 is responsible for leucocyte mobility
    d   IgA activates the alternative pathway
    e   C7 deficiency is found in Raynaud's phenomenon

13 HLA DR3 is associated with:
    a   systemic lupus erythematosus
    b   Behçet's disease
    c   Sjögren's syndrome
    d   myasthenia gravis
    e   frozen shoulder

14 Immunoglobulin:
    a   D has little antibody activity
    b   G is able to cross the placenta
    c   A is present in the circulation in dimeric form
    d   M is produced early in primary response to an antigen
    e   E is able to activate complement

15 Raised IgE levels are found in:
    a   coeliac disease
    b   rheumatoid arthritis
    c   Hodgkin's disease
    d   pulmonary haemosiderosis
    e   systemic lupus erythematosus

16 The following are found in the Wiskott-Aldrich syndrome:
    a   raised IgM levels
    b   defective cell-mediated immunity
    c   autosomal dominant inheritance
    d   lymphoma as a terminal event
    e   thrombocytosis

17 In ankylosing spondylitis:
    a   morning stiffness is associated
    b   symptoms improve with exercise
    c   the peripheral joints are spared
    d   plantar fasciitis occurs
    e   renal impairment may occur

(Answers overleaf)

12 a c d e
The complement system involves at least nine different proteins. Activation is triggered by immunoglobulins and antibody-antigen interactions. The ultimate effect of activation is destruction and lysis of bacteria. C2 mediates kinin activity and C1qrs induces vascular permeability.

13 a c d
HLA DR3 is associated with Addison's disease, SLE, Sjögren's syndrome, chronic hepatitis, coeliac disease, Graves' disease and myasthenia gravis. Behcet's syndrome is associated with HLA B12 and 'frozen shoulder' is associated with HLA B27.

14 a b d
IgA provides protection at mucous membranes. In serum it is monomeric and in secretory form, dimeric. IgE is the 'reaginic' antibody and is able to bind to mast cells. This antibody is responsible for acute anaphylaxis. IgG is the main plasma immunoglobulin and is the only one which is able to cross the placenta. Complement activation can only occur with IgG and IgM.

15 a c d
Raised IgE levels are seen in atopic states, parasitic infestations, Hodgkin's disease, coeliac disease, nephrotic syndrome and bronchopulmonary aspergillosis.

16 b d
This is a condition due to abnormal lymphocyte function leading to eczema and abscesses. It is X-linked and reflects pathology of platelet and lymphocyte plasma membrane. There is thrombocytopenia and raised IgE levels. Death is usually in the second decade from B cell lymphoma or cerebral haemorrhage.

17 a b d
Ankylosing spondylitis is associated with an insidious onset, M>F, morning stiffness and improvement with exercise. HLA B27, Reiter's syndrome and psoriasis are associated. Constitutional symptoms including fatigue and weight loss are not uncommon. Complications include aortic incompetence, AV conduction defects, respiratory insufficiency, cauda equina lesions and uveitis. Treatment consists of physiotherapy and anti-inflammatory drugs. Radiotherapy is no longer used due to the increased incidence of leukaemia amongst those previously treated in this way.

18 The following conditions can present with bone/joint symptoms:
   a motor neurone disease
   b carcinoma of the pancreas
   c atrial myxoma
   d hypoparathyroidism
   e chronic leukaemia

19 The following findings in a patient make it more likely that she has rheumatoid arthritis than systemic lupus erythematosus:
   a normal serum complement levels
   b lymphopenia
   c synovitis
   d reduced glucose in pleural fluid
   e bone erosions

20 Pseudogout is caused by:
   a hypoparathyroidism
   b Wilson's disease
   c haemochromatosis
   d ochronosis
   e osteoarthrosis

(Answers overleaf)

18 a b c d e
There are many conditions which have rheumatological presentations including infections (hepatitis A and B, rubella and brucellosis), metabolic disease (haemochromatosis, Wilson's disease and amyloidosis), lung cancer, breast cancer, sickle cell anaemia and inflammatory bowel disease, to list but a few.

19 d e
Complement may be normal/high in RA and normal/low in SLE; lymphopenia is more a feature of SLE and synovitis may occur in both.

20 b c d
Pseudogout (pyrophosphate arthropathy) is caused by a variety of conditions including pernicious anaemia, ochronosis, haemochromatosis, Wilson's disease, RA, hyperparathyroidism and hypomagnesaemia.

17. Statistics

1 The following statements are true:
   a the mean is the middle observation
   b the mode is the most frequently occurring value
   c the arithmetic mean is the sum of all the observations multiplied by the number of observations
   d the geometric mean is always less than the arithmetic mean
   e the standard deviation is the square of the variance

2 The following are examples of non-parametric statistical tests:
   a Wilcoxon rank sum
   b Spearman rank correlation
   c Student 't' test
   d Mann Whitney 'U' test
   e Chi squared

3 Using Chi squared:
   a numbers must first be converted to percentages
   b two populations may be compared
   c the test relates to frequencies of the occurrence of individuals in the various categories of one or more variables
   d the degree of freedom can be calculated by the formula: (No. columns − 1) + (No. rows − 1)
   e the larger the value of Chi squared the greater the similarity between observed and expected frequencies

(Answers overleaf)

1 b d
The mean is the sum of all the observations divided by the number of observations. The geometric mean is the antilogarithm of the arithmetic mean of logarithmic values.

2 a b d
Non-parametric tests are used when no assumptions are made about a distribution, when there is non-normality of data, and when data are measured by a ranked scale. Student's 't' test and Chi squared are parametric tests.

3 b c
This test relates to frequencies of the occurrence of individuals in the categories of one or more variables. The numbers are *not* converted to percentages and the degrees of freedom can be calculated by:

[No. columns − 1] × [No. rows − 1]

The larger the value of Chi squared the greater the *disparity* between observed and expected frequencies.

4 The following statistical definitions are correct:
   a   a type II error is one in which a hypothesis is not rejected when it should have been
   b   the significance level is the probability associated with a type I error
   c   a negatively skewed distribution has a longer tail extending towards the higher values of the variable
   d   the geometric mean is the antilogarithm of the arithmetic mean of log values
   e   in an ordered set 25% of observations lie below the first, above the third and between successive quartiles

5 In linear regression:
   a   correlation relates to the interdependence of two variables
   b   regression is concerned with the dependence of one variable on another
   c   a value for r (correlation coefficient) of +1 always means complete correlation
   d r is dimensionless
   e   sampling distribution of r is normal

(Answers overleaf)

4 a b d e
A type I error occurs when a hypothesis is rejected when it is true and a type II error occurs when a hypothesis is not rejected when it is false.

5 a b c d
When talking about correlation the interdependence between x and y are quantified. A value for $r = 0$ means there is no linear relationship between x and y and a value of $+1$ means there is a perfect linear relationship; r is dimensionless and the sampling distribution of r is not normal.

Recommended Reading

The following method of working is a personal one and worked for me. I divide my books into three main groups. The first is the large textbook (e.g. *The Oxford textbook of medicine*) which I refer to when in doubt or if there is something I do not understand and wish to read in depth. The MRCP candidate should not spend a great deal of time reading these since, in my opinion, they do not help you get through the exam! The second type of book is the monograph devoted to one particular topic. These are worth reading in some detail and are useful for making your own revision notes. The third type of book I use is the 'list' book and there are several of these on the market at present. This type of book is useful for supplementing your notes (which should read like lists anyway) and provides the sort of 'small print' required in MRCP Part 1.

LARGE TEXTS

British Medical Association/Pharmaceutical Society of Great Britain 1988 British national formulary

Isselbacher K J et al 1980 Harrison's principles of internal medicine. McGraw Hill, New York

Weatherall, D J, Ledingham J G G, Warrell D A (eds) 1987 The Oxford textbook of medicine, 2nd edn. Oxford University Press, Oxford

LIST BOOKS

Burton J L 1988 Aids to postgraduate medicine, 5th edn. Churchill Livingstone, Edinburgh

Epstein R J 1985 Medicine for examinations: a streamlined approach to revision. Churchill Livingstone, Edinburgh

Gabriel R, Gabriel C M 1988 Medical lists for examinations, 2nd edn. Butterworths, London

Lim Y L 1981 Revision notes in clinical medicine. Pitman Publishing Ltd, London

Margulies D M, Thaler M S 1983 The physician's book of lists. Churchill Livingstone, Edinburgh

READING FOR SPECIFIC AREAS

Basic sciences
Ellis H 1983 Clinical anatomy: a revision and applied anatomy for clinical students, 7th edn. Blackwell Scientific Publications, Oxford
Scratcherd T 1981 Aids to physiology. Churchill Livingstone, Edinburgh

Cardiology
Dawkins K D 1987 Manual of cardiology. Churchill Livingstone, Edinburgh
Julian D G 1988 Cardiology, 5th edn. Balliere Tindall, London
Turner R W D, Gold R G 1984 Auscultation of the heart, 5th edn. Churchill Livingstone, Edinburgh

Dermatology
MacKie R M 1986 Clinical dermatology: an illustrated textbook, 2nd edn. Oxford University Press, Oxford

Endocrine/metabolic
Muirhead N, Catto G R D 1986 Aids to fluid and electrolyte balance. Churchill Livingstone, Edinburgh
Reynolds D J, Freeman H G M 1986 Aids to clinical chemistry. Churchill Livingstone, Edinburgh
Zilva J F, Pannall P R 1984 Clinical chemistry in diagnosis and treatment, 4th edn. Lloyd-Luke, London

Gastroenterology
There are four issues of Medicine International dealing with this subject and these are worth a read.
Elias E, Hawkins C 1985 Lecture notes on gastroenterology. Blackwell, Oxford

Genetics
Weatherall D J 1985 The new genetics and clinical practice, 2nd edn. Oxford Medical Publications, Oxford

Haematology
Child J A 1982 Aids to clinical haematology. Churchill Livingstone, Edinburgh
Hoffbrand A V, Lewis S M 1981 Postgraduate haematology, 2nd edn. Heinemann, London

Infectious disease
The Medicine International series is particularly good on infectious diseases and I would recommend reading and making notes from these.

RECOMMENDED READING

Neurology
Lindsay K W, Bone I, Callander R 1986 Neurology and neurosurgery illustrated. Churchill Livingstone, Edinburgh

Ophthalmology
Perkins E S, Hansell P, Marsh R J 1986 An atlas of diseases of the eye, 3rd edn. Churchill Livingstone, Edinburgh

Paediatrics
Hull D, Johnston D I 1987 Essential paediatrics, 2nd edn. Churchill Livingstone, Edinburgh

Pharmacology
The BNF provides an excellent source of lists such as prescribing in pregnancy, liver disease and so on.
Rogers H, Spector R 1986 Aids to pharmacology, 2nd edn. Churchill Livingstone, Edinburgh

Renal disease
Brown C B 1985 Manual of renal disease. Churchill Livingstone, Edinburgh

Respiratory medicine
The section on respiratory medicine in the OTM is excellent and well worth reviewing and making notes from, as are the sections on respiratory diseases in Medicine International.
Mitchell D 1986 Respiratory medicine revision: MCQs, case histories and data interpretation. Churchill Livingstone, Edinburgh

Rheumatology/Immunology
Medicine International deals with both these subjects fairly well and I would recommend reading these.

Statistics
Petrie A 1987 Lecture notes on medical statistics, 2nd edn. Blackwell Scientific Publications, Oxford

Index

The first number refers to the page and the number in parentheses refers to the question number.

Abetalipoproteinaemia, 73 (5)
Abscess, amoebic liver, 45 (12)
Achalasia, 41 (1)
Acid phosphatase, raised serum level, 71 (2)
Acrodermatitis enteropathica, 93 (15)
Acromegaly, 37 (15)
Acute tubular necrosis, see Tubular necrosis acute
Acquired immune deficiency syndrome (AIDS) virus, 63 (6)
ACTH, see Adrenocorticotrophic hormone
Acute intermittent porphyria, see Porphyria
Addison's disease, 37 (14)
ADH, see Antidiuretic hormone
Adrenal hyperplasia, congenital, 37 (13)
Adrenocorticotrophic hormone, 3 (5)
Adverse drug reactions, 97 (6)
Aldosterone, 35 (7)
Alopecia, 31 (9)
Alport's syndrome, 111 (18)
Alveolar-capillary block, 115 (7)
Anaemia, immune haemolytic and drugs, 57 (19)
Anaphylactoid purpura, see Henoch Schönlein purpura
Anion gap, 75 (16), 107 (9)
Ankle jerk, 83 (15)
Ankylosing spondylitis, 125 (17)
Anorexia nervosa, 75 (15)
Anthrax, 65 (13)
Anti-arrhythmic drugs, 23 (20)
Antibacterial drugs, 63 (5)
Antibiotics, batericidal, 95 (1)
Anticancer drugs, 99 (16)
Antidiuretic hormone, 105 (1)
  inappropriate, 33 (5)
Antithrombin III deficiency, 55 (14)

Antitrypsin deficiency, (α_1), 119 (17)
Ascites, 13 (34)
Atropine, side effects, 95 (2)
Autosomal dominant inheritance, 49 (1)

Behcet's syndrome, 121 (2)
Benign intracranial hypertension, 85 (17)
Bile acids, functions, 1 (4)
Bilirubin, presence in urine, 15 (39)
Blood pressure,
  afterload reducers, 21 (16)
  regulation, 7 (18)
Breast-feeding, and drugs, 101 (19), 123 (11)
Bronchiolitis, 89 (4)
Bronchoalveolar lavage, 119 (19)
Bronchoconstrictors, 97 (7)
Brucellosis, 65 (14)
Bundle branch block, right, 25 (26)

Café au lait spots, 29 (1)
Calcitonin, 13 (35)
Carbon monoxide poisoning, 115 (9)
Carcinoembryonic antigen (CEA), 53 (9)
Carcinoid tumour, 47 (18)
Carcinoma
  hepatocellular, 41 (2)
  stomach, 47 (19)
  thyroid, 35 (6)
Cardiac rupture, 17 (1)
Cardiomyopathy, restrictive, 25 (28)
Central nervous system,
  neurotransmitters, 5 (11)
Cerebrospinal fluid, 79 (1), 85 (20)
Chest x-ray, basal changes, 113 (1)
Chi squared, 129 (3)
Chlamydia, 69 (24)
Cholera toxin, 61 (3)

INDEX

Cholesterol, 21 (14)
Chronic active hepatitis, see Hepatitis, chronic active
Chronic granulomatous disease, 55 (17)
Cimetidine, 97 (8)
Cirrhosis, primary biliary, 43 (5)
Colitis,
  ulcerative, 45 (13)
  pseudomembranous, 43 (9)
Complement, 107 (7), 125 (12)
Congenital adrenal hyperplasia, 37 (13)
Convulsions, neonatal, 91 (6)
Cranial nerve, tenth, 5 (10)
Creatine kinase, 5 (13), 5 (14)
Crohn's disease, 43 (10), 45 (13)
Cryoglobulinaemia, 121 (1)
Cryptococcal infection 67 (17)
Cushing's disease, 37 (16)

Developmental milestones, 89 (1)
Deviation, right axis, 25 (24)
Diabetes insipidus, 11 (29)
Dialysis, peritoneal, 7 (17)
Diaphragm, 3 (8)
Dimorphic blood film, 51 (4)
Diphosphoglyceric acid (2,3-DPG), 53 (7)
Diuretics, loop, 97 (9)
Dopamine agonists, 39 (17)
Dusts, fibrogenic, 113 (2)
Dysphasia, 81 (10)
Dystrophy,
  facioscapulohumeral, 81 (8)
  myotonic, 81 (7)

Echocardiography, 17 (2)
Eosinophilic alveolar reactions, 115 (6)
Eruption
  fixed drug, 29 (4)
  photosensitive, 31 (7)
Erythema multiforme, 29 (3)
Erythrocyte sedimentation rate (ESR), 55 (13)
Erythropoietin, 13 (33)
Exercise testing, 21 (12)
Exophthalmos, 33 (2)

Fabry's disease, 123 (10)
Fanconi syndrome, 77 (18)
Fasciculation, muscle, 79 (4)
Ferritin, 9 (27)
Fibrosing alveolitis, 115 (5)
First heart sound, see Heart sound, first
Fourth heart sound see Heart sound, fourth
Friedreich's ataxia, 81 (9)

Gallstones, 43 (7)
Gastrin, release, 7 (20)
Gastrinoma, see Zollinger-Ellison syndrome
Glandular fever, 63 (9)
Glucagon, 37 (12)
Glucose intolerance, 35 (8)
Glucose-6-phosphate dehydrogense (G6PD) deficiency, 57 (22)
Gluten-free diet, 43 (8)
Goitrogens, 101 (20)
Goodpasture's syndrome, 119 (18)
Gout, childhood, 121 (5)
Growth hormone, 35 (9), 99 (12)
Gynaecomastia, 33 (1)

Haemochromatosis, 73 (9)
Haemodialysis, 7 (17), 107 (8)
Haemoglobin A2, 57 (21)
Heart,
  anatomy, 9 (22)
  block, first degree, 17 (4)
  disease, congenital cyanotic, 27 (30)
  sound,
    first, 19 (11)
    fourth, 23 (22)
    second, 19 (6)
Henoch Schönlein purpura, 93 (12)
Hepatic granulomata, 43 (6)
Hepatitis,
  chronic active, 45 (15)
  surface antigen, 45 (11)
Hepatolenticular degeneration, see Wilson's disease
Hirsutism, 99 (17)
Histamine, 9 (24)
Histiocytosis X, 91 (8)
Homocystinuria, 71 (4)
Hormone, growth, 35 (9), 99 (12)
Human leucocyte antigen (HLA) DR3, 125 (13)
Hyperbilirubinaemia, 45 (14)
Hypercalcaemia, 77 (19)
Hyperlipidaemia, 77 (17)
Hypertension,
  benign intracranial, 85 (17)
  primary pulmonary, 21 (17)
Hypertrophy, right ventricle, 21 (13)
Hypoglycaemia, recurrent, 33 (3)
Hypoglycaemic drugs, 33 (4)

INDEX 139

Hypokalaemia, 11 (28), 109 (15)
Hypokalaemic periodic paralysis, 85 (19)
Hypomagnesaemia, 11 (32)
Hyponatraemia, 109 (16)
Hypoparathyroidism, neonatal, 91 (11)
Hypophosphataemia, 75 (11)
Hypopituitarism, 35 (11)
Hyposplenism, 55 (12)
Hypothermia, 75 (12)

Immunoglobulin, 125 (14)
   E, raised levels, 125 (15)
Incubation periods, 61 (1)
Insulin, 99 (14)
Interval
   PR, 19 (9)
   QT, 19 (5), 95 (5)
Iron
   absorption, 13 (37)
   metabolism, 51 (3)
Isoniazid toxicity, 69 (25)

Jaundice, cholestatic, 47 (17)
Jugular venous pressure, 25 (27)

Kala-azar, 67 (20)
Kartagener's syndrome, 113 (3)
Kidney, large, 105 (4)
Klinefelter's syndrome, 49 (2)

Lateral medullary syndrome, 83 (14)
Left atrial myxoma, see Myxoma, left atrial
Legionnaire's disease, 65 (11)
Leprosy, 67 (21)
Leptospirosis, 67 (18)
Leukaemia, acute, 53 (8)
Linear regression, 131 (5)
Lumbosacral plexus, see Plexus, lumbosacral
Lung disease, restrictive, 117 (12)
Lymphocytes, T versus B, 15 (40)
Lymphocytosis, 59 (24)

Macrocytosis, 13 (36)
Magnesium, renal excretion, 5 (12)
Malignancy, inherited conditions predisposing to, 49 (3)
Malignant hyperpyrexia, 49 (4)
Measles, 63 (10)
Mediastinal masses, anterior, 117 (14)
Melioidosis, 67 (19)
Methaemoglobinaemia, 55 (15)

Monoamine oxidase inhibitors, 95 (3)
Monocytosis, 53 (11)
Multiple sclerosis, 81 (9)
Muscarinic receptors, 9 (23)
Myasthenia gravis, 83 (11)
Myxoma, left atrial, 23 (21)

Nails, blue, 31 (8)
Nephroblastoma, 91 (9)
Nephrotic syndrome, 107 (6)
Nerve,
   radial, 3 (7)
   ulnar, 7 (21), 81 (5)
   vagus, 5 (10)
Neuropathy,
   autonomic, 79 (2)
   motor, 85 (18)
Neutropenia, 63 (8)
Non-parametric statistical tests, 129 (2)
Norwalk virus, 47 (20)
Nucleotidase, 5', 75 (13)

Obstructive sleep apnoea, 117 (13)
Oral contraceptives, 97 (11)
Osteomalacia, 73 (8)
Osteoporosis, 75 (14)
Ovarian tumours, and androgen secretion, 39 (18)
Oxygen dissociation curve, 3 (6)

Paget's disease of bone, 71 (1)
Pancreatitis, acute, 41 (3)
Pancytopenia, 51 (5)
Papillitis, 87 (5)
Papilloedema, 87 (5)
Paraproteinaemia, 5 (15)
Parathyroid hormone, 11 (30)
Parietal lobe lesions, 85 (16)
Parkinsonian features, diseases with, 81 (6)
Pemphigoid, 29 (2)
Pemphigus, 29 (2)
Penicillamine, 121 (4)
Pericarditis, constrictive, 21 (15)
Phaeochromocytoma, 39 (20)
Phenytoin, side effects, 95 (4)
Phosphate reabsorption, 9 (26)
Platelet count, elevated, 57 (20)
Pleural effusions, 117 (16)
Plexus, lumbosacral, 3 (9)
Pneumoconiosis, 113 (4)
Pneumothorax, 117 (10)
Polyarteritis nodosa, 23 (18)
Polyarthritis, acute, 123 (9)

INDEX

Polycythaemia rubra vera, 53 (6)
Porphyria
  acute intermittent, 73 (6)
  and drugs, 77 (20), 101 (23)
Prader-Willi syndrome, 93 (13)
Pregnancy,
  cardiovascular system, 23 (23)
  drugs safe, 101 (18)
Premalignant skin lesions, 31 (10)
Primary biliary cirrhosis, see
    Cirrhosis, primary biliary
Primary pulmonary hypertension,
  see Hypertension, primary
PR interval, see Interval, PR
Prostaglandins, metabolism, 7 (16)
Proteins,
  plasma, 1 (2)
  serum which rise with tissue
    damage, 73 (10)
Proteinuria, 11 (31)
Pseudogout, 127 (20)
Pseudohypoparathyroidism, 35 (10)
PTH, see Parathyroid hormone
Pulmonary
  alveolar proteinosis, 115 (8)
  vasculature, prominent, 23 (19)
Pupil, large, 87 (1)
Pyloric stenosis, 91 (7)
Pyuria, 107 (11)

QT interval, see interval, QT

Radial nerve, palsy, see Nerve, radial
Receptors,
  muscarinic, 9 (23)
Red blood cells, nucleated, 59 (25)
Reiter's syndrome, 121 (2)
Relapsing polychondritis, 123 (7)
R wave, dominant in V1, 19 (10)
Renal
  failure,
    chronic, 107 (10)
    drugs to avoid, 101 (21)
    haemodialysis, 7 (17), 107 (8)
  papillary necrosis, 105 (2)
  phosphate absorption, 9 (26)
  stones, radiolucent, 105 (3)
  tubular acidosis (RTA), 71 (3), 105 (5)
Renin, 109 (14)
Respiration, pre- and post-natal, 9 (25)
Respiratory distress syndrome of newborn, 89 (3)
Retinitis pigmentosa, 87 (4)
Retinopathy, diabetic, 87 (2)

Retroperitoneal fibrosis, 109 (13)
Reye's syndrome, 89 (5)
Rheumatic fever, 25 (29)
Rheumatoid arthritis,
  pleural effusions, 123 (8)
  poor prognosis, 121 (3)
  versus SLE, 127 (19)
Right axis deviation, see Deviation, right axis
Right bundle branch block, see Bundle branch block, right:
Right ventricular hypertrophy, see Hypertrophy, right ventricle

Salmonella, food poisoning, 65 (15)
Sarcoidosis, 117 (15), 119 (20)
Second heart sound, see Heart sound, second
Short stature, 93 (14)
Sideroblasts in bone marrow, 57 (23)
Sodium, homeostasis, 1 (1)
Somatomedin, 7 (19)
Spastic paraparesis, 79 (3)
Splenectomy, blood film post-, 53 (10)
Splenomegaly, 13 (38)
Subacute combined degeneration, 83 (13)
Syphilis, false-positive serology, 69 (22)
Syringomyelia, 83 (12)
Systemic lupus erythematosus (SLE)
  versus rheumatoid arthritis, 127 (19)
Systemic sclerosis, 123 (6)

Tachycardia, ventricular, versus supraventricular, 25 (25)
Target cells, 51 (1)
Theophylline clearance, 117 (11)
Thrombosis, retinal vein, 87 (3)
Thyroid binding globulin, 39 (19), 99 (13)
Toxocara, 69 (23)
Transplacental infections, 89 (2)
Trichinosis, 65 (16)
Tricyclic antidepressants. ECG changes, 17 (3)
Tubular necrosis, acute, 111 (19)
Turner's syndrome, 49 (5)
Typhoid fever, 61 (4)

Ulceration, legs, 29 (5)
Ulcerative colitis, 45 (13)
Ulnar nerve, see Nerve, ulnar
Uraemia, prerenal, 111 (19)

Urine,
  acidification, 97 (10)
  red, 109 (12)
  strongly acid, 109 (17)

Vaccines, live, 61 (2)
Vagus nerve, *see* Nerve, vagus
Vasculature, prominent pulmonary, 23 (19)
Venous hum, 19 (7)
Viruses, DNA, 63 (7)
Vitamins, 1 (3)
Vitiligo, 31 (6)

Von Willebrand's disease, 57 (18)

Waldenström's macroglobulinaemia, 55 (16)
Warfarin, potentiation, 99 (15)
Whooping cough, 65 (12)
Wilson's disease, 45 (16), 73 (7)
Wiskott-Aldrich syndrome, 125 (16)
Wolff-Parkinson-White syndrome, 19 (8)

Zollinger-Ellison syndrome, 41 (4)

111.50 net

OFU 201190